Handbook for attention deficit hyperactivity disorder in adults

CW00971678

Handbook for attention deficit hyperactivity disorder in adults

UK Adult ADHD Network (UKAAN)
Philip Asherson (UKAAN President)
Susan Young (UKAAN Vice President)
Marios Adamou
Blanca Bolea
David Coghill
Gisli Gudjonsson
James Kustow
Ulrich Müller
Mark Pitts
Johannes Thome

www.ukaan.org

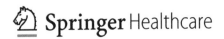 Springer Healthcare

Published by Springer Healthcare Ltd, 236 Gray's Inn Road, London, WC1X 8HB, UK.

www.springerhealthcare.com

© 2013 Springer Healthcare, a part of Springer Science+Business Media.

All rights reserved. No part of this publication may be reproduced, stored in a retrieval system or transmitted in any form or by any means electronic, mechanical, photocopying, recording or otherwise without the prior written permission of the copyright holder.

British Library Cataloguing-in-Publication Data.

A catalogue record for this book is available from the British Library.

ISBN 978-1-908517-50-0

Although every effort has been made to ensure that drug doses and other information are presented accurately in this publication, the ultimate responsibility rests with the prescribing physician. Neither the publisher nor the authors can be held responsible for errors or for any consequences arising from the use of the information contained herein. Any product mentioned in this publication should be used in accordance with the prescribing information prepared by the manufacturers. No claims or endorsements are made for any drug or compound at present under clinical investigation.

Project editor: Katrina Dorn
Designer: Joe Harvey
Artworker: Sissan Mollerfors
Production: Marina Maher
Printed in Great Britain by Latimer Trend & Company Ltd.

Contents

Author biographies		**ix**
Acknowledgments		**xv**

1	**Introduction to attention deficit hyperactivity disorder**	**1**
	References	3

2	**Definition of attention deficit hyperactivity disorder in adults**	**5**
	Diagnostic criteria	5
	Changes to Diagnostic and Stastical Manual of Mental Disorders	9
	Age of onset	9
	Subthreshold cases	13
	Comorbid pervasive developmental disorder	14
	Defining impairment in attention deficit hyperactivity disorder	14
	References	16

3	**The scientific basis of attention deficit hyperactivity disorder in adults**	**17**
	Prevalence of attention deficit hyperactivity disorder	17
	Validity of the diagnostic construct	19
	Main validating criteria	20
	Etiology	24
	Environmental risks	27
	Cognitive processes	30
	Neuroimaging and electrophysiology	30
	Electrophysiological investigations	33
	References	36

4 Diagnostic assessment of attention deficit hyperactivity disorder in adults 41

Key principles 41

Diagnosing attention deficit hyperactivity disorder in adults 42

Diagnostic protocol 46

References 53

5 Neuropsychological assessment 55

Neuropsychological tests 56

Case studies 60

References 64

6 Comorbid symptoms, syndromes, and disorders 65

Clinical implications 65

Sources of comorbid symptoms, syndromes, and disorders 66

Core symptoms not listed within current operational criteria 66

Neurodevelopmental disorders and overlapping etiological influences 68

Attention deficit hyperactivity disorder as a risk factor for other
mental health disorders and behavioral problems 69

Diagnosis and treatment of attention deficit hyperactivity disorder and
comorbid disorders 71

References 82

7 Pharmacological treatments 87

Choice of drug therapy 87

Drug prescribing 89

Methylphenidate 93

Amphetamines 102

Atomoxetine 108

Bupropion 114

Other substances 116

Combination treatment 118

References 119

8 Psychological treatments   **123**

NICE clinical guidelines   124

Cognitive behavioral therapy   125

Dialectical behavioral therapy   132

Coaching   133

Summary   134

References   134

9 Attention deficit hyperactivity disorder during pregnancy   **137**

General considerations   138

Treatment   138

Maternal behavior during pregnancy   140

Attention deficit hyperactivity disorder treatment and breastfeeding   141

References   142

10 Attention deficit hyperactivity disorder and the criminal justice system   **145**

Attention deficit hyperactivity disorder and crime   145

Post-conviction   149

Treatment of offenders with attention deficit hyperactivity disorder   149

Summary   150

References   151

11 Service provision for adults with attention deficit hyperactivity disorder   **153**

Service populations   154

Costs of attention deficit hyperactivity disorder   155

Trends in service delivery   156

Pathways of care: a value-based approach   158

Service structure and determinants of service provision   160

Summary   165

References   165

Author biographies

UKAAN

The UK Adult ADHD Network (UKAAN) was established in March 2009 to provide support, education, research and training for mental health professionals working with adults with attention deficit hyperactivity disorder (ADHD). UKAAN was founded by a group of experienced mental health specialists who run clinical services for adults with ADHD within the National Health Service. The network was established in response to UK guidelines from the National Institute of Health and Clinical Excellence (NICE, 2008) and the British Association for Psychopharmacology (Nutt et al, 2007), which, for the first time, gave evidence-based guidance on the need to diagnose and treat ADHD in adults as well as in children; and in response to the relative lack of training and support in this area for professionals working within adult mental health services. The aim of UKAAN is to support clinicians in the development of clinical services for adults with ADHD.

Contributors

Marios Adamou (MD, MA, MSc, LL.M , MBA, PhD, PGCE, MRCPsych, CMgr MCMI, DOccMed, FHEA, FRSA, FRSPH) is a consultant psychiatrist for the Service for Adults with ADHD in South West Yorkshire Partnership NHS Foundation Trust. He has been working in the area of Service Development for over 8 years having set up services for patients with bipolar disorder and adult ADHD. Dr Adamou has postgraduate qualifications in history, law, business administration, medical education, and occupational medicine. His publications include practical manuals on setting up Services for patients with bipolar disorder and adult ADHD. He has extensive research experience in multinational studies and has been the principal investigator in Phase III studies for adults with ADHD. His main research interests are in employment and medico-legal issues of adults with ADHD.

Professor Philip Asherson (MB, BS, MRCPsych, PhD) is Professor of Molecular Psychiatry at the MRC Social, Genetic and Developmental Psychiatry centre at the Institute of Psychiatry, King's College London, and consultant psychiatrist at the Maudsley Hospital. He earned his medical degree from The Royal London Hospital and his doctoral degree from the University of Wales. He was an MRC Clinical Research Fellow in the Department of Psychological Medicine and Institute of Medical Genetics at the University Of Wales College Of Medicine in Cardiff, where he worked on molecular genetic studies of schizophrenia. His current work focuses on clinical, quantitative genetic, and molecular genetic studies of ADHD across the lifespan. He has contributed to the development of mental health services for adults with ADHD in the UK. He is President of the UK Adult ADHD Network (www.UKAAN.org), a professional network that aims to support clinical research, education, and service provision for adults with ADHD. He was a member of the guideline development group for the National Institute of Health and Clinical Excellence (NICE) and contributed to published guidelines from NICE, the British Association of Psychopharmacology and the European Network Adult ADHD consensus paper. Current research includes follow-up studies of ADHD from childhood to adulthood, investigation of mood instability and emotional regulation in ADHD, treatment of ADHD in young offenders, defining the psychopathology of ADHD; and quantitative and molecular genetic studies of ADHD and associated cognitive-neurophysiological endophenotypes. He has published more than 220 peer reviewed articles, including guideline documents on diagnosis and treatment of ADHD in adults.

Blanca Bolea (MD, Esp. Psiq (Spain), Dip. Estudios Avanzados) is currently a consultant psychiatrist at Trincay Medical Services, Cayman Islands. She graduated from the University of Zaragoza in Spain and underwent specialist training in Madrid. She subsequently worked at the Maudsley Hospital (London, UK) and in the Hopital Cantonale de Marsans (Switzerland). She joined the psychopharmacology unit at Bristol University in 2005 and worked in the psychopharmacology clinic under the supervision of Professor David Nutt, with whom Dr Bolea founded the Bristol Adult ADHD Clinic in 2007. Current research interests include neurosteroids and their relationship with ADHD, and environmental influences in pregnancy related to ADHD outcomes in children.

David Coghill (MB ChB, MRCPsych) is a reader in child and adolescent psychiatry, Department of Psychiatry, University of Dundee. Dr Coghill is head of the Developmental Research Group within the Department of Psychiatry, University of Dundee. This group has a particular interest in the neuropsychopharmacology of ADHD and has recently completed a large study into the effects of stimulant medication on neuropsychological functioning in ADHD. Dr Coghill's other areas of interest are the interactions between basic and clinical sciences in ADHD and disruptive behavior disorders, psychopharmacological treatments in child psychiatry and the use of evidence based approaches to care within real world settings. In his clinical practice, he is joint clinical lead for the developmental neuropsychiatry team in Tayside and maintains a special interest in forensic child and adolescent psychiatry.

Professor Gisli Gudjonsson (CBE, BSc, MSc, PhD, FBPsS) is an Emeritus Professor of Forensic Psychology at the Institute of Psychiatry, King's College London, and an honorary consultant in clinical and forensic psychologist at Broadmoor Hospital. He is a Chartered Clinical and Forensic Psychologist and a Fellow of the British Psychological Society. He is a registered practitioner with the Health Professions Council (HPC). In 2009 his professional body, the British Psychological Society, granted him a Lifetime Achievement Award for his exceptional and sustained contribution to the practice of psychology. He was awarded The European Association of Psychology and Law (EAPL) Life Time Achievement Award for 2012 and was appointed a Commander of the Order of the British Empire (CBE) in the Queen's Birthday 2011 Honours List for services to clinical psychology. He has published extensively in the areas of forensic psychology, including violence, sexual offending, psychogenic amnesia, stress, psychological vulnerability, suggestibility, false confession, police interviewing, attention deficit hyperactivity disorder, and false/recovered memories.

James Kustow (BMedSci, BMBS, MRCPsych) is a consultant psychiatrist and medical lead for a new 'complex care' service in Enfield. The service, quite unique in its approach and ethos, places far more emphasis on psychotherapeutic intervention and proactive episodes of care than the traditional community psychiatry model. Dr Kustow has a specialist clinical expertise working with adult ADHD, both in terms of its diagnosis and medical management, and the development of comprehensive psychosocial interventions by working with and building on people's strengths to develop effective strategies to promote balanced, healthy living and positive relationships. He has worked alongside Dr Leon Rozewicz in local adult ADHD service in Edgware, one of the few London-based NHS services of its kind. Dr Kustow is the latest member of the UKAAN executive board and he also sits on the Training Committee and was instrumental in the development of UKAAN's national training program. He has a variety of other interests including liaison psychiatry, traumatic memory and its various manifestations, and somatically-focused psychological interventions including eye movement desensitization and reprocessing (EMDR). Dr Kustow is the founder of the 'Marrow' charity, affiliated to 'The Anthony Nolan Trust,' which is based in UK medical schools, as well as in six other countries. This student-run medical organization provides a third of the bone marrow donor registrations in the UK.

Ulrich Müller (MD [Dr. med., Univ. Würzburg], PhD [Dr. med. habil., Univ. Leipzig]), is a senior university lecturer at the Department of Psychiatry, University of Cambridge, and Honorary Consultant Psychiatrist with Cambridge University Hospitals NHS Foundation Trust and Cambridgeshire and Peterborough Foundation NHS Trust (CPFT). Dr Ulrich is a consultant psychiatrist for the Rehabilitation and Recovery team in Huntingdon England. He is director of the Adult ADHD Research Clinic at Addenbrooke's Hospital in Cambridge and senior clinical collaborator of the ADHD/Impulsive-Compulsive Disorders cluster at the Behavioural and Clinical Neuroscience Institute (BCNI). Ulrich is a board member of the UK Adult ADHD Network (UKAAN) and consults for several adult ADHD service development projects in East Anglia. Before Dr Ulrich arrived in Cambridge in 2003, he trained in psychiatry, psychotherapy, neurological rehabilitation, and cognitive neuroscience in Germany (Würzburg, Munich, and Leipzig). His research focuses on adult ADHD and cognitive-enhancing medication. He has published more than 100 articles in scientific journals and book chapters and is a regular speaker at national training events and international scientific conferences.

Mark Pitts (BSc [Hons], Psychology and Nursing) is the clinical nurse specialist at the Adult ADHD Service, which is an outpatient clinic based at the Maudsley Hospital, and one of a number of national specialist services offered by the South London and Maudsley NHS Foundation Trust. The Adult ADHD Service is a national service specializing in the assessments and treatment of adults with ADHD, and was the first such service in the United Kingdom. Nurse Pitts role predominantly focuses on providing follow-up reviews to monitor patients' responses to medication in conjunction with the consultant psychiatrist, and advising patients and their local clinicians on titration to the optimum medication dosage, as well as assisting in the initial assessment process, and overseeing the day-to-day running of the service. Nurse Pitts has degrees in psychology and learning disability nursing, and worked for 5 years in a national low-secure service for people with a mild/borderline learning disability at the Bethlem Royal Hospital in London prior to taking up his current position in 2005. His clinical interests are in the assessment of ADHD in adults, pharmacological treatment and follow-up, and the development of adult ADHD services. He also sits on the steering committee of the UK ADHD Nursing Network, whose main aim is to provide a regular conference aimed at nurses working in this specialism.

Johannes Thome (MD, PhD) is head of the Department of Psychiatry and Psychotherapy at the University of Rostock, Germany, where aside from treatment of mental illness, he wishes to create a new center for molecular psychiatry. Professor Thome studied medicine, philosophy, and social psychology and obtained his MD and PhD degrees from Saarland University, Germany. He completed his training in psychiatry at the University of Wurzburg, Germany, and then became Postdoctoral Associate at the Division of Molecular Psychiatry at Yale School of Medicine (USA).

After 2 years of intensive and successful research in the area of molecular psychiatry and psychopharmacology, he worked as consultant psychiatrist and senior lecturer at the Central Institute of Mental Health Mannheim, University of Heidelberg, Germany. From 2004–2011, he was Chair of Psychiatry at the Institute of Life Sciences, Swansea University in Wales.

Susan Young (BSc [Hons], DClinPsy, PhD) is a clinical senior lecturer in forensic clinical psychology in the Department of Forensic and Neurodevelopmental Sciences at the Institute of Psychiatry, King's College London. She is programme leader of the MSc program in clinical forensic psychology at King's College London Institute of Psychiatry and an honorary consultant clinical and forensic psychologist at the high secure Broadmoor Hospital. Dr Young has extensive clinical experience in the assessment and treatment of youths and adults with ADHD and in the assessment and treatment of offenders with mental illness and/or mental disorder. Previously, she was employed as a clinical neuropsychologist at the Maudsley Hospital, where she set up and developed the neuropsychology service at the first adult ADHD service in the United Kingdom. Dr Young participated in the British Association of Psychopharmacology Consensus Meeting (2007) to develop guidelines for management of transition for ADHD adolescents to adult services. She was a member of the National Institute for Health and Clinical Excellence (NICE) ADHD Clinical Guideline Development Group (2008); her main contributions being discussions on psychological treatment of children and adults with ADHD, transition and the provision of expert guidance on the clinical procedures and services required for the diagnosis and treatment of ADHD in adults. Dr Young has acted as a consultant regarding ADHD service development in the UK, Iceland and the Republic of Ireland, in addition to consulting on UK and European ADHD advisory boards sponsored by industry. Dr Young has published articles in scientific journals and books, three psychological intervention programmes and has authored two books. Dr Young is currently leading a research group, supported by the Department of Health, which aims to develop projects that will establish the evidence base on ADHD and offenders and approaches to their management in the criminal justice system.

Acknowledgments

We thank all UKAAN members for their support of this initiative. In particular, the educational committee (Muhammad Arif, Sally Cubbin, Stephanos Maltezos, Clodagh Murphy, Leon Rozewicz) who have all made important contributions to the delivery of training on diagnosis and treatment to mental health professionals in the UK. Special thanks to Susan Dunn Morua of AADDUK (www.aadduk.org) and Andrea Bilbow of ADDISS (www.addiss.co.uk) for supporting the development of clinical services and user support groups in the UK and representing the perspective of children, adolescents, and adults with ADHD. Also, thanks to David Nutt for his support of UKAAN and review of the final draft of this handbook. Finally, the co-authors would all like to thank Sue Curtis for keeping us all on track and her constant energy and enthusiasm for this project.

Chapter 1

Introduction to attention deficit hyperactivity disorder

Attention deficit hyperactivity disorder (ADHD) is a common mental health disorder that affects an estimated 3.6% of children [1] and 2.5% of adults [2,3] in the UK. The disorder is well established in childhood, with rapid service development since the mid-1990s. As a result, almost all regions of the UK have child and adolescent mental health or pediatric services with expertise in the diagnosis and treatment of ADHD in young people. Depending on the severity of the condition and co-occurring mental health or psychosocial problems, these young people generally will receive medical, social, and educational interventions. Follow-up studies of children with ADHD indicate that approximately 15% retain the full ADHD diagnosis at age 25, and a further 50% remain in partial remission, with persistence of some symptoms associated with significant impairments [4]. Yet until recently, adult services have been poorly developed in the UK and other parts of Europe, despite the known impact that ADHD has on adult mental health.

The National Institute of Health and Clinical Excellence (NICE) guidelines published in 2009 represent a milestone in the development of effective clinical services for patients with ADHD across the lifespan [5]. The NICE guideline committee systematically reviewed available evidence and provided comprehensive guidelines for the clinical management of ADHD, including, for the first time both the preschool and post-adolescent years. The guideline clearly delineates a disorder that can be devastating to individuals and their families at all ages and

UKAAN, *Handbook for Attention Deficit Hyperactivity Disorder in Adults*, DOI: 10.1007/978-1-908517-79-1_1, © Springer Healthcare 2013

provides a clear recommendation for the establishment of local adult mental health services for patients with ADHD. Similar recommendations have also been made in a consensus review from the British Association of Psychopharmacology published in 2006 [6] and, more recently, in a consensus statement on ADHD in adults from the European Network Adult ADHD [7].

These developments will come as no surprise to the large majority of child and adolescent psychiatrists who have followed many patients with ADHD from initial diagnosis and treatment into the adult years. Many practitioners are well aware of the persistence of the disorder into adulthood and have been demanding transitional arrangements for their patients for some time. Furthermore, because of the high familial risk of ADHD, they are also aware of the high proportion of parents of children with ADHD who present with similar problems.

Yet, until recently, many primary and secondary care physicians have failed to recognize the disorder in adults. The reasons for this are not entirely clear, but may relate to the traditional separation of child and adolescent psychiatry from adult psychiatry. This has led to the independent development of diagnostic classificatory systems for childhood developmental disorders and adult-onset disorders, and it is only in recent years that a lifespan perspective has more readily been considered. This is particularly a problem in understanding the underlying problems in chronic trait-like conditions, such as personality disorders, which in some cases have their origins in neurodevelopmental and childhood-onset behavioral disorders, and the impact of childhood-onset neurodevelopmental disorders such as ADHD, on adult psychopathology. Some adult psychiatrists are also unwilling to diagnose and treat ADHD in adults because they are unfamiliar with the drugs used to treat ADHD and concerned about their controlled status and their supposed addictive properties.

Another difference is the traditional use of informant assessments of behavior as the main source of clinical diagnosis in child and adolescent psychiatry, in contrast to the focus on the mental state examination and self-report to investigate psychiatric disorders in adults. This has led to expectations among adult psychiatrists that disorders such as ADHD are primarily defined by behavior, neglecting the subjective experiences (phenomenology) of ADHD subjects. An example of this would be the patient who describes being distracted by unfocused thought processes and feeling that they are 'always on the go' and that flit from one topic to another, a phenomena that can be both distressing and impairing to adults with ADHD.

The recognition of ADHD as an adult disorder means that clinicians in both primary and secondary care require specialist training to diagnose and manage the disorder beyond the childhood years. New clinics for adults with ADHD are being established in many regions of the UK and other parts of Europe, to provide clinical services for those transitioning from adolescent to adult services, as well as for patients with ADHD that are diagnosed for the first time in adulthood.

This book provides an essential outline and step-by-step guide to the process of recognition, diagnosis, treatment, and long-term support for adults with ADHD. The book was written by the executive committee for the UK Adult ADHD Network (UKAAN: www.ukaan.org), a group of UK-based adult mental health professionals with many years of experience working with adults with ADHD. The contents of this book are based on guidelines from NICE, the British Association of Psychopharmacology, and international organizations such as the Canadian ADHD Resource Alliance (CADDRA) and European Network Adult ADHD, which provide evidence-based views of ADHD diagnosis and clinical management. We hope that this clinical handbook will provide a set of protocols that are easy to follow in clinical practice and will lead to better recognition and treatment, improvements in impairment and associated comorbid conditions, and an increase in overall quality of life for adults with ADHD.

References

1   Ford T, Goodman R, Meltzer H. The British child and adolescent mental health survey 1999: the prevalence of DSM-IV disorders. *J Am Acad Child Adolesc Psychiatry*. 2003;42:1203-1211.
2   Fayyad J, De Graaf R, Kessler R, et al. Cross-national prevalence and correlates of adult attention-deficit hyperactivity disorder. *Br J Psychiatry*. 2007;190:402-409.
3   Simon V, Czobor P, Balint S, et al. Prevalence and correlates of adult attention-deficit hyperactivity disorder: meta-analysis. *Br J Psychiatry*. 2009;194:204-211.
4   Faraone, SV, Biederman J, Mick E. The age-dependent decline of attention deficit hyperactivity disorder: a meta-analysis of follow-up studies. *Psychol Med*. 2006;36:159-165.

5   National Institute for Health and Clinical Excellence (NICE). Attention deficit hyperactivity
    disorder: The NICE guideline on diagnosis and management of ADHD in children, young
    people, and adults. NICE website. 2008; www.nice.org.uk/CG072. Accessed April 13, 2012.
6   Nutt DJ, Fone K, Asherson P, et al. Evidence-based guidelines for management of attention-deficit/
    hyperactivity disorder in adolescents in transition to adult services and in adults:
    recommendations from the British Association for Psychopharmacology. *J Psychopharmacol*.
    2007;21:1041.
7   Kooij SJJ, Bejerot S, Blackwell A, et al. European consensus statement on diagnosis and
    treatment of adult ADHD: The European Network Adult ADHD. *BMC Psychiatry*. 2010;10:67.

Chapter 2

Definition of attention deficit hyperactivity disorder in adults

Attention deficit hyperactivity disorder (ADHD) is a clinical syndrome defined in the *Diagnostic and Statistical Manual of Mental Disorders (DSM-IV)* [1] by high levels of hyperactive, impulsive, and inattentive behaviors that begin during early childhood, are persistent over time, pervasive across situations, and lead to clinically significant impairments. Current DSM-IV criteria use a list of 18 symptom items, with 9 for hyperactivity-impulsivity and 9 for inattention [2]. Under the International Classification of Disease (ICD-10) classification system endorsed by the World Health Organization [3], the condition is referred to as hyperkinetic disorder, which is a more restricted definition of the disorder, describing a severe subgroup of patients with the combined subtype of ADHD.

Diagnostic criteria
Diagnostic and Statistical Manual of Mental Disorders
DSM-IV diagnosis is made if six or more items in either the inattentive or hyperactive-impulsive domains are present, leading to three subtypes (criterion A) [2]:

- inattentive type of ADHD;
- hyperactive type of ADHD;
- combined type of ADHD.

Impairing symptoms should emerge before the age of 7 years (criterion B), with some impairment in more than one setting (criterion C), and affecting social, occupational, or academic performance (criterion D). Finally, the disorder should not be caused by another condition (criterion E).

UKAAN, *Handbook for Attention Deficit Hyperactivity Disorder in Adults*, DOI: 10.1007/978-1-908517-79-1_2,
© Springer Healthcare 2013

In adults, some of the symptoms that are present in childhood will have remitted or modified with developmental age, so that some patients who are still impaired by symptoms of ADHD may no longer meet the full diagnostic criteria. Yet persistence of some symptoms with a significant impairment means that they may still require treatment and fulfill the DSM-IV criteria for 'ADHD in partial remission.' Table 2.1 describes the formal DSM-IV criteria for ADHD.

Diagnostic and Statistical Manual of Mental Disorders: diagnostic criteria for attention deficit hyperactivity disorder

A. Either (1) or (2):

1. Six or more of the following symptoms of inattention have persisted for at least six months to a degree that is maladaptive and inconsistent with the developmental level:

Inattention

- often fails to give close attention to details or makes careless mistakes in schoolwork, work, or other activities
- often has difficulty sustaining attention in tasks or play activities
- often does not seem to listen when spoken to directly
- often does not follow through on instructions and fails to finish schoolwork, chores, or duties in the workplace (not due to oppositional behavior or failure of comprehension)
- often has difficulty organizing tasks and activities
- often avoids, dislikes, or is reluctant to engage in tasks that require sustained mental effort (eg, schoolwork or homework)
- often loses things necessary for tasks or activities at school or at home (eg, toys, pencils, books, assignments)
- is often easily distracted by extraneous stimuli
- is often forgetful in daily activities

2. Six or more of the following symptoms of hyperactivity–impulsivity have persisted for at least 6 months to a degree that is maladaptive and inconsistent with the developmental level:

Hyperactivity

- often fidgets with hands or feet or squirms in seat
- often leaves seat in classroom or in other situations in which remaining seated is expected;
- often runs about or climbs excessively in situations in which it is inappropriate (in adolescents or adults, may be limited to subjective feelings of restlessness)
- often has difficulty playing or engaging in leisure activities quietly
- often talks excessively
- is often 'on the go' or often acts as if 'driven by a motor'

Impulsivity

- often has difficulty awaiting turn in games or group situations
- often 'blurts out' answers to questions before they have been completed
- often interrupts or intrudes on others (eg, butts in to other children's games)

B. Some hyperactive–impulsive or inattentive symptoms that cause impairment were present before the age of 7 years

Table 2.1 *Diagnostic and Statistical Manual of Mental Disorders:* diagnostic criteria for attention deficit hyperactivity disorder (continues opposite).

Diagnostic and Statistical Manual of Mental Disorders: diagnostic criteria for attention deficit hyperactivity disorder (continued)

C. Some impairment from the symptoms is present in two or more settings (eg, at school, work, and/or at home)

D. There is clear evidence of clinically significant impairment in social, academic, and/or occupational functioning

E. The symptoms do not occur exclusively during the course of a pervasive developmental disorder, schizophrenia, or other psychotic disorder, and are not better accounted for by another mental disorder (eg, mood disorder, anxiety disorder, dissociative disorder, or other personality disorder)

Based on these criteria, three types of ADHD have been identified:

1. *Combined type:* if both criteria 1A and 1B are met for the past 6 months
2. *Predominantly inattentive type:* if criterion 1A is met, but criterion 1B is not met for the past 6 months
3. *Predominantly hyperactive-impulsive type:* if criterion 1B is met, but criterion 1A is not met for the past 6 months

Broader subtypes of ADHD:

In partial remission: this subtype applies to individuals (especially adolescents and adults) who currently have symptoms that no longer meet full criteria

ADHD not otherwise specified: this subtype includes disorders with prominent inattention or hyperactivity-impulsivity that do not meet criteria for ADHD. Examples include:

- individuals who meet criteria for ADHD but whose age of onset is 7 years or older
- individuals with clinically significant impairment who present with inattention and whose symptom pattern does not meet the full diagnostic criteria for ADHD, but have a behavioral pattern marked by sluggishness, daydreaming, and hypoactivity

Table 2.1 *Diagnostic and Statistical Manual of Mental Disorders:* **diagnostic criteria for attention deficit hyperactivity disorder (continued).** ADHD, attention deficit hyperactivity disorder; DSM-IV; Diagnostic and Statistical Manual of Mental Disorders, 4th Edition; Reprinted with permission from American Psychiatric Association [2].

International classification of disease: hyperkinetic disorder

Under the tenth edition of the International Classification of Disease (ICD-10) system [3] (Table 2.2), the condition is referred to as hyperkinetic disorder. This is considered a more restricted definition of ADHD that delineates a severe form of the Combined Type as defined in DSM-IV. NICE guidelines (2009) recommend that children and adolescents with hyperkinetic disorder require immediate treatment with medication [4].

One limitation of the ICD-10 criteria is the hierarchical rule for comorbid disorders, which results in ADHD being excluded as a diagnosis if it occurs in the presence of other common adult mental health disorders. Since ADHD in adults is commonly accompanied by such conditions (eg, depression), this limits the usefulness of the ICD-10 criteria in clinical practice.

ICD-10 criteria and recommendations for use in clinical practice

Demonstrable abnormality of attention, activity and impulsivity at home, for the age and developmental level of the child, as evidenced by (1), (2), and (3):

1. Patient demonstrates at least three of the following attention problems:
   A. short duration of spontaneous activities
   B. often leaving play activities unfinished
   C. over-frequent changes between activities
   D. undue lack of persistence at tasks set by adults
   E. unduly high distractibility during study (homework or reading assignment)

2. Patient also demonstrates at least three of the following activity problems:
   A. very often runs about or climbs excessively in situations where it is inappropriate
   B. seems unable to remain still
   C. markedly excessive fidgeting and wriggling during spontaneous activities
   D. markedly excessive activity in situations expecting relative stillness (eg, mealtimes, travel, visiting, church)
   E. often leaves seat in classroom or other situations when remaining seated is expected; often has difficulty playing quietly

3. Patient also demonstrates at least one of the following impulsivity problems:
   A. often has difficulty awaiting turns in games or group situations;
   B. often interrupts or intrudes on others (eg, interrupts others' conversations or games);
   C. often blurts out answers to questions before questions have been completed

Demonstrable abnormality of attention and activity at school or nursery (if applicable), for the age and developmental level of the child, as evidenced by both (1) and (2):

1. Patient demonstrates at least two of the following attention problems:
   A. undue lack of persistence at tasks
   B. unduly high distractibility (ie, often orienting toward extrinsic stimuli)
   C. overfrequent changes between activities when choice is allowed
   D. excessively short duration of play activities

2. Patient also demonstrates at least three of the following activity problems:
   A. continuous (or almost continuous) and excessive motor restlessness (eg, running, jumping in situations allowing free activity)
   B. markedly excessive fidgeting and wriggling in structured situations
   C. excessive levels of off-task activity during tasks
   D. unduly often out of seat when required to be sitting
   E. often has difficulty playing quietly

Directly observed abnormality of attention or activity. This must be excessive for the child's age and developmental level. The evidence may be any of the following:

1. direct observation of the criteria above (ie, not solely the report of parent or teacher);
2. observation of abnormal levels of motor activity, or off-task behavior, or lack of persistence in activities in a setting outside home or school (eg, in a clinic or laboratory)
3. significant impairment of performance on psychometric tests of attention

Does not meet criteria for pervasive developmental disorder, mania, depressive, or anxiety disorder

Onset before the age of 7 years

Duration of at least 6 months

IQ above 50

Table 2.2 ICD-10 criteria and recommendations for use in clinical practice. ICD-10, Tenth edition of the International Classification of Disease; Adapted with permission from World Health Organization [3].

Changes to Diagnostic and Stastical Manual of Mental Disorders

Despite the widespread use of the DSM-IV criteria, several criticisms have been leveled at them, including the lack of developmental consistency in adults [4]. For example, criteria referring to 'climbing' and 'playing quietly' cannot easily be applied outside childhood. Another criticism is the threshold of six symptoms, which may be excessively high when applied to adults. Suggested changes to the DSM-IV criteria include:

- an increase in the permitted age of onset;
- the addition of age-adjusted descriptions of ADHD symptoms that are suitable for use in adults;
- the inclusion of behaviors that reflect deficits of executive functions and emotional lability;
- an adjustment of symptom threshold;
- to allow comorbidity with pervasive developmental disorders;
- replace term 'clinical subtypes' with 'clinical presentations'.

Thus, there are numerous changes that have been considered for the forthcoming DSM-V (Table 2.3).

Age of onset

Although the onset of ADHD symptoms is often seen in early childhood, this is not always the case; a significant group have impairing ADHD symptoms that start later in life. Comparisons of patients that fulfill

Proposed changes in the fifth edition of the Diagnostic and Statistical Manual of Mental Disorders
• Change the age of onset from onset of impairing symptoms by age 7 years to onset of symptoms by age 12 years
• Change the three subtypes to three current presentations
• Add a fourth presentation for restrictive inattentive
• Change the examples in the items – without changing the exact wording of the DSM-IV items – to accommodate a lifespan relevance of each symptom and to improve clarity
• Remove pervasive developmental disorders from the exclusion criteria
• Modify the preamble (A1 and A2) to indicate that information must be obtained from two different informants (eg, parents and teachers for children and third party/significant other for adults), whenever possible
• Adjust the age cut-off point for diagnosis in adults (still under consideration)

Table 2.3 **Proposed changes in the fifth edition of the Diagnostic and Statistical Manual of Mental Disorders.**

criteria for ADHD with an age of onset beyond 7 years of age have shown them to be similar to those with an earlier age of onset, with similar predictions for clinical outcome, treatment response, and risk of associated disorders [4,6,7].

In some cases, ADHD symptoms may be less severe in early childhood, with impairments emerging during the secondary school years when there is more demand on self-control of behavior and academic performance. In some cases, ADHD may not emerge as an impairing problem until the young person leaves home and is expected to organize his or her own life. Additionally, both a high cognitive ability and a structured child environment can contribute to masking the problems associated with ADHD in some high-functioning individuals. A further problem is that adults tend to report the onset of ADHD symptoms an average of 5 years later than the actual age at which the symptoms started [8], perhaps related to difficulty in recalling behavior before the age of 12 years.

In the majority of cases, impairing symptoms from ADHD are apparent by the age of 12 years, and this is the criterion that has been adopted by many specialists in the field. We therefore recommend that the age of onset criteria should be altered to symptoms that start before the age of 12 years or by early adolescence. The requirement for onset of impairment in childhood should be dismissed, so long as current impairment can be shown to be the direct result of ADHD symptoms. These changes are expected to be applied to the DSM-V criteria.

Age-adjusted criteria for symptoms in adults

Symptom items for ADHD within the DSM-IV are not adjusted for developmental changes that occur in all people as they grow older. The symptoms persist but their typical presentation changes. Examples of age-adjusted descriptions have been provided in an earlier publication and are reproduced in Table 2.4 [9] and are also incorporated into the Diagnostic Interview for Adult ADHD (DIVA) (see Appendix G).

Descriptions of ADHD symptoms need to take into account the developmental age of individuals. Examples of age-appropriate descriptions of symptoms for adults are expected to be included in DSM-V [10].

Age-adjusted attention deficit hyperactivity disorder symptoms for use with adults

Inattention

☐ *Often fails to give close attention to detail.* Has difficulty remembering where they put things. At work, this may lead to costly errors. Tasks that require detail and are considered tedious (eg, income tax returns) become very stressful. This may include overly 'perfectionist'-like and rigid behavior, and needing too much time for tasks involving details in order to prevent forgetting any of them

☐ *Often has difficulty sustaining attention.* Inability to complete routine tasks (eg, tidying a room or mowing the lawn) without forgetting the objective and starting something else. Inability to sustain sufficient attention to read a book that is not of special interest, although there is no reading disorder. Inability to keep accounts, write letters, or pay bills. Attention often can be sustained during exciting, new, or interesting activities (eg, using internet, chatting, computer games). This does not exclude the criterion when boring activities are not completed

☐ *Often does not seem to listen when spoken to.* Receive complaints that they do not listen or that it is difficult to gain their attention. Even where they appear to have heard, they forget what was said and do not follow through. These complaints reflect a sense that they are 'not always in the room', 'not all there', or 'not tuned in'

☐ *Fails to follow through on instructions and complete tasks.* Adults with ADHD may observe difficulty in following other people's instructions (eg, inability to read or follow instructions in a manual for appliances). Failure to keep commitments undertaken (eg, work around the house)

☐ *Difficulty organizing tasks or activities.* Recurrent errors (eg, lateness, missed appointments, missing critical deadlines). Sometimes a deficit in this area is seen in the amount of delegation to others such as secretary at work or spouse at home

☐ *Avoids or dislikes sustained mental effort.* Puts off tasks such as responding to letters, completing tax returns, organizing old papers, paying bills, establishing a will. These adults often complain of procrastination

☐ *Often loses things needed for tasks* (eg, misplacing purse, wallet, keys, assignments from work, where car is parked, tools, and even children!)

☐ *Easily distracted by extraneous stimuli.* Subjectively experience distractibility and describe ways in which they try to overcome this. This may include listening to white noise, multi-tasking, requiring absolute quiet, or creating an emergency to achieve adequate states of arousal to complete tasks. Often has many projects going simultaneously and has trouble with completion of tasks

☐ *Forgetful in daily activities.* May complain of memory problems. For example, a patient may head out to the supermarket with a list of things, but end up coming home having failed to complete their tasks or having purchased something other than what they intended to buy

Hyperactivity

☐ *Fidgets with hands or feet.* This item may be observed, but it is also useful to ask patient about this. Fidgeting may include picking their fingers, shaking knees, tapping hands or feet, and changing position. Fidgeting is most likely to be observed while the patient is waiting in the waiting area of the clinic

☐ *Leaves seat in situations in which remaining seated is usual.* Adults may be restless. For example, patients become frustrated with dinners out in restaurants or are unable to sit during conversations, meetings, and conferences. This may also manifest as a strong internal feeling of restlessness when waiting

Table 2.4 Age-adjusted attention deficit hyperactivity disorder symptoms for use with adults (continues overleaf).

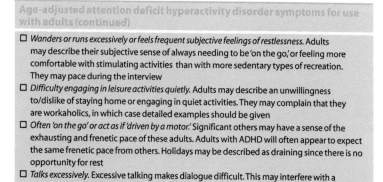

Age-adjusted attention deficit hyperactivity disorder symptoms for use with adults (continued)

☐ *Wanders or runs excessively or feels frequent subjective feelings of restlessness.* Adults may describe their subjective sense of always needing to be 'on the go', or feeling more comfortable with stimulating activities than with more sedentary types of recreation. They may pace during the interview

☐ *Difficulty engaging in leisure activities quietly.* Adults may describe an unwillingness to/dislike of staying home or engaging in quiet activities. They may complain that they are workaholics, in which case detailed examples should be given

☐ *Often 'on the go' or act as if 'driven by a motor.'* Significant others may have a sense of the exhausting and frenetic pace of these adults. Adults with ADHD will often appear to expect the same frenetic pace from others. Holidays may be described as draining since there is no opportunity for rest

☐ *Talks excessively.* Excessive talking makes dialogue difficult. This may interfere with a spouse's sense of 'being heard' or achieving intimacy. This chatter may be experienced as nagging and may interfere with normal social interactions. Clowning around, repartee, or other means of dominating conversations may mask an inability to engage in give-and-take conversation

Impulsivity

☐ *Answers before questions have been completed.* This will usually be observed during the interview. This may also be experienced by probands as a subjective sense of other people talking too slowly and finding it difficult to wait for them to finish. Tendency to say what comes to mind without considering timing or appropriateness

☐ *Difficulty waiting in turn.* Adults find it difficult to wait for others to finish tasks at their own pace, such as children. They may feel irritated waiting in line or in a restaurant and may be aware of their own intense efforts to force themselves to wait. Some adults compensate for this by carrying something to do at all times

☐ *Interrupts or intrudes on others.* This is most often experienced by adults as social ineptness at social gatherings or even with close friends. An example might be inability to watch others struggle with a task (such as trying to open a door with a key) without jumping in to try the task for themselves

Table 2.4 Age-adjusted attention deficit hyperactivity disorder symptoms for use with adults (continued). ADHD, attention deficit hyperactivity disorder. Reproduced with permission from Asherson [9].

Behaviors that reflect deficits in executive function

Some experts conceptualize ADHD symptoms as primarily a deficit of executive functions. While this is not always reflected in neuropsychological testing of executive functions, impairments are usually seen in the way that people with ADHD manage daily tasks [8,11]. Such impairments include difficulties with self-organization, timekeeping, losing things, attention span, emotion regulation, sustaining effort, and alertness. Table 2.5 lists some of the behaviors that reflect difficulties with executive function.

Behaviors reflecting difficulties with executive functions are commonly seen in adults with ADHD, either reflecting core ADHD symptoms or

Activation	Organizing, prioritizing, and initiating work
Focus	Focusing, sustaining, and shifting attention to tasks
Effort	Regulating alertness, sustaining effort, and processing speed
Emotion	Managing frustration and regulating emotions
Memory	Utilizing working memory and accessing recall
Action	Monitoring and self-regulating activities

Table 2.5 Behavioral domains in adults with attention deficit hyperactivity disorder that are proposed to reflect difficulties with executive function. Reproduced with permission from Brown et al [11].

commonly associated features of the disorder. Future editions of the operational diagnostic criteria may adopt some of these symptoms as either core or commonly associated features of ADHD.

Subthreshold cases

Follow-up studies of children with ADHD and cross-sectional epidemiological studies have found that, as adults, individuals with ADHD retain significant levels of impairment linked to persistence of ADHD symptoms, albeit symptoms are sometimes at subthreshold levels [12–15].

As a response to this situation, it has been proposed that the number of symptoms required for a diagnosis of ADHD in adulthood should be reduced from the current six or more (as in DSM-IV) to four or more [12], as long as the symptoms are clearly linked to impairments and began during childhood or early adolescence. Application of this revised criterion would be in line with the DSM-IV category of ADHD in partial remission, and would ensure that people with significant impairments from persistence of ADHD symptoms in adulthood would be diagnosed and treated. Despite these considerations it is not certain that the recommended change in symptom threshold will be adopted in the DSM-V [10].

When assessing the diagnosis of ADHD in adults, clinicians should aim to establish the diagnosis in childhood and track the persistence of symptoms through to the time of assessment. Where it is not possible to obtain detailed accounts of symptoms and behaviors from before the age of 12 years, clinical judgment will need to be used to decide whether the current symptoms reflect persistence of ADHD from childhood or early adolescence.

Comorbid pervasive developmental disorder

Both the DSM-IV and ICD-10 criteria state that ADHD or hyperkinetic disorder should not be diagnosed in the presence of a pervasive developmental disorder (eg, autism spectrum disorder; ASD). Yet in clinical practice, the ADHD syndrome is commonly found to be comorbid with ASD.

In practice, ADHD and ASD are often diagnosed together and co-occurrence of both disorders will be possible in DSM-V [10]. The 2008 NICE guidelines already clarify that it is possible to have both disorders, and that the diagnosis of ADHD should be made on the basis of the core syndrome, regardless of comorbidity [4].

Clinical presentations

The traditional inattentive, hyperactive-impulsive and combined subtypes of ADHD have been found to be developmentally unstable. For example, it is not unusual to see someone meet clinical criteria for the hyperactive-impulsive subtype during early childhood, combined-type ADHD during middle childhood and early adolescence, and the inattentive subtype as young adults. This reflects normal developmental changes seen in the wider population but may also reflect poor sensitivity of the items for hyperactive-impulsive symptoms as adults mature and manage some of their symptoms better. Because of the instability of the clinical subtypes, DSM-V will refer to these as clinical presentations with the expectation that they will often change throughout the lifetime of an individual with ADHD [10].

Defining impairment in attention deficit hyperactivity disorder

The presence of impairment linked to the symptoms of ADHD is critical to the diagnostic construct of ADHD as a mental health disorder. When considering the diagnosis of ADHD, symptoms are defined on the basis of being extreme for the developmental age of the person and leading to clinically significant impairments. We can think of ADHD as reflecting the extreme and impairing tail of continuous traits of inattentive and hyperactive-impulsive symptoms and behaviors that can also lead to the development of comorbid disorders. In this respect, ADHD is similar to conditions such as obesity, high blood pressure, anxiety, and depression.

Defining the level of impairment that is required for a diagnosis of ADHD is to some extent arbitrary and will depend on cultural and social expectations. Yet we can provide basic 'common-sense' guidelines to ensure that ADHD diagnosis is restricted to those who present with a significant mental health disorder. In exactly the same way, we need to decide, for example, whether a patient presenting with an anxiety disorder or depression – both common syndromes experienced by most people at some time – are severe enough to warrant medical or psychological interventions. The 2008 NICE guidelines provide recommendations on the level of impairment required for the diagnosis of ADHD (Table 2.6) [4].

The range of impairments seen in ADHD is very broad and encompasses people who barely function to people who maintain themselves in relatively high-powered jobs. ADHD impairments are not only defined by cross-sectional severity of functional impairments, but also by the

Defining impairment in attention deficit hyperactivity disorder

Impairment in ADHD should have the following features:

- Specialist professional intervention is required to avoid long-term adverse implications of the impairment (as well as problems in the short and medium term)
- Impairment is pervasive, occurs in multiple settings, and is of at least moderate severity
- Symptoms relating to the impairment should cause problems in at least two domains. Domains of impairment include:
  – personal distress from ADHD symptoms
  – lowered self esteem (usually related to functional impairment)
  – problems with social interactions and relationships
  – impaired function in academic, employment, and daily activities
  – increase in driving accidents and risk-taking behavior
  – development of comorbid psychiatric syndromes and behavioral problems
- Significant impairment should not be considered if the impact of ADHD symptoms is restricted to academic performance alone without a moderate-to-severe impact in other domains. A diagnosis of ADHD should not be applied to justify the use of stimulant medication for the sole use of increasing academic performance

Table 2.6 Defining impairment in attention deficit hyperactivity disorder. ADHD, attention deficit hyperactivity disorder. Adapted with permission from NICE [4].

chronicity of the disorder and the long-term impact on emotional and social aspects of a patient's everyday life. We all experience poor concentration and respond impulsively at times (eg, when we are tired or 'hungover'). However, patients with ADHD experience such difficulties most of the time and to an extent that impairs function in daily life and causes subjective distress. The chronicity of the disorder and the impact on function from childhood through to adulthood is an important aspect of impairment, with cumulative effects on self esteem, mental well-being, and health-related quality of life.

References

1   American Psychiatric Association. *Diagnostic and Statistical Manual of Mental Disorders*. 4th edition. Washington DC: American Psychiatric Association; 1994.

2   American Psychiatric Association. *Diagnostic and Statistical Manual of Mental Disorders*. 4th edition, text revision. Washington, DC: American Psychiatric Association; 2000.

3   World Health Organisation. *The ICD-10 Classification of Mental and Behavioural Disorders*. Geneva: World Health Organisation; 2002. www.who.int/classifications/icd/en/GRNBOOK.pdf. Accessed August 25, 2012.

4   National Institute for Health and Clinical Excellence (NICE). Attention deficit hyperactivity disorder: *The NICE Guideline on Diagnosis and Management of ADHD in Children, Young People, and Adults*. NICE website. www.nice.org.uk/CG072. Accessed August 25, 2012.

5   McGough JJ, Barkley RA. Diagnostic controversies in adult attention deficit hyperactivity disorder. *Am J Psychiatry*. 2004;161:1948-1956.

6   Applegate B, Lahey BB, Hart EL, et al. Validity of the age-of onset criterion for ADHD: a report from the DSM-IV field trials. *J Am Acad Child Adolesc Psychiatry*. 1997;36:1211-1221.

7   Faraone S V, Biederman J, Spencer T, et al. Diagnosing adult attention deficit hyperactivity disorder: are late onset and subthreshold diagnoses valid? *Am J Psychiatry*. 2006;163:1720-1729.

8   Barkley R, Murphy KR, Fischer M. *ADHD in Adults: What the Science Says*. New York, NY: Guilford Press; 2007.

9   Asherson, P. Clinical assessment and treatment of attention deficit hyperactivity disorder in adults. *Expert Rev Neurother*. 2005;5:525-539.

10 American Psychiatric Association. DSM-5 development. A 06 Attention deficit disorder/hyperactivity disorder. APA website. www.dsm5.org/ProposedRevision/Pages/proposedrevision.aspx?rid=383. Accessed August 25, 2012.

11 Brown TE. Executive functions and attention deficit hyperactivity disorder: implications of two conflicting views. *Int J Disability, Development Education*. 2006;53:35-46.

12 Kooij JJ, Buitelaar JK, van den Oord EJ, et al. Internal and external validity of attention-deficit hyperactivity disorder in a population-based sample of adults. *Psychol Med*. 2005;35:817-827.

13 Faraone SV, Biederman J, Mick E. The age-dependent decline of attention deficit hyperactivity disorder: a meta-analysis of follow-up studies. *Psychol Med*. 2006;36:159-165.

14 Fayyad J, De Graaf R, Kessler R, et al. Cross-national prevalence and correlates of adult attention-deficit hyperactivity disorder. *Br J Psychiatry*. 2007;190:402-409.

15 Kessler RC, Adler L, Barkley R, et al. The prevalence and correlates of adult ADHD in the United States: results from the National Comorbidity Survey Replication. *Am J Psychiatry*. 2006;163:716-723.

The scientific basis of attention deficit hyperactivity disorder in adults

Prevalence of attention deficit hyperactivity disorder

Prevalence in children

There are a wide range of prevalence rates for attention deficit hyperactivity disorder (ADHD) cited in the world literature, with recent estimates converging on a figure of 5% during the childhood years [1]. The most recent figures from the British Child and Adolescent Mental Health Survey in the UK estimate a rate of 3.6% in boys and 0.9% in girls for any subtype of ADHD (Table 3.1) [2].

	Gender		Age				
	Male (%)	Female (%)	5–7 years (%)	8–10 years (%)	11–12 years (%)	13–15 years (%)	Average (%)
All ADHD subtypes	3.6	0.9	1.9	2.5	2.6	2.1	2.2
ADHD combined type	2.3	0.5	1.5	1.5	1.6	1.1	1.4
ADHD inattentive type	1.0	0.3	0.2	0.9	0.7	0.9	0.7
ADHD hyperactive-impulsive type	0.3	<0.1	0.2	0.1	0.3	0.1	0.2

Table 3.1 Estimated prevalence of childhood attention deficit hyperactivity disorder in the UK by gender and age. ADHD, attention deficit hyperactivity disorder. Reproduced with permission from Ford et al [2].

UKAAN, *Handbook for Attention Deficit Hyperactivity Disorder in Adults*, DOI: 10.1007/978-1-908517-79-1_3, © Springer Healthcare 2013

Prevalence in adults

In adults, prevalence estimates range from 2.5 to 4.3% (Figure 3.1) [3–5]. These figures are in line with follow-up studies of children with ADHD that estimate that around two-thirds of patients with ADHD in childhood retain impairing levels of ADHD symptoms by 25 years of age [6]. Recent data on prescription rates of drug treatments for ADHD in the UK suggest that there is a marked reduction in the numbers of individuals treated beyond 18 years of age, which does not reflect what is known about the natural course of the disorder and is far in excess of that predicted by remission rates [7].

The wide range in prevalence rates cited in the literature almost certainly reflects differences in the way that ADHD symptoms have been measured and the way that operational criteria have been applied across the different studies. Symptom thresholds for ADHD are difficult to define with any degree of certainty because they lie on a continuum in the general population, which means there is no natural boundary between affected and unaffected individuals. Definitions of ADHD also depend critically on the way that impairment and pervasiveness across situations are defined. This was demonstrated in a study of 7- and 8-year-olds from Newcastle,

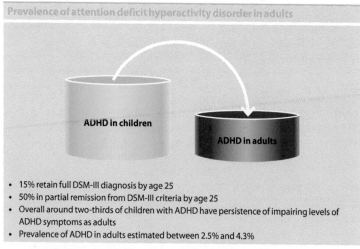

Prevalence of attention deficit hyperactivity disorder in adults

ADHD in children

ADHD in adults

- 15% retain full DSM-III diagnosis by age 25
- 50% in partial remission from DSM-III criteria by age 25
- Overall around two-thirds of children with ADHD have persistence of impairing levels of ADHD symptoms as adults
- Prevalence of ADHD in adults estimated between 2.5% and 4.3%

Figure 3.1 Prevalence of attention deficit hyperactivity disorder in adults. ADHD, attention deficit hyperactivity disorder; DSM, Diagnostic and Statistical Manual of Mental Disorders. Data taken from Fayyad et al [3], Kessler et al [4], Simon et al [5] and Faraone et al [9].

which found a prevalence of 11.1% when symptom count alone was used to define the disorder, 6.7% when an impairment score (Children's Global Assessment of Functioning Scale [C-GAS] <71) was applied, 4.2% with a more severe impairment threshold (C-GAS <61), and only 1.4% when pervasiveness was also taken into account [8].

Another reason for differences in reported prevalence rates within the literature on ADHD in adults, relates to different ways in which the *Diagnostic and Statistical Manual of Mental Disorders (DSM-IV)* criterion of "some symptoms and impairments occurring before the age of 7 years" has been applied. This criterion has generally been interpreted to mean that some symptoms in either domain are allowed during childhood (eg, two symptoms before the age of 7 years has been used as a criterion, but not necessarily meeting full ADHD criteria in childhood or adolescence), so long as there are six or more symptoms in the 6 months prior to the adult assessment [3,4]. Others have used stricter criteria reguiring that the full diagnosis was met during childhood [9,10].

Validity of the diagnostic construct

Diagnosis and treatment of ADHD in adults is now well-established, yet the validity of the diagnostic construct continues to be questioned [11,12]. While reliability for operationally defined ADHD has been established, validity remains an important issue, particularly because of symptom overlap with other common mental health disorders and difficulties in drawing clear distinctions between ADHD and the normal range of attention, activity, and impulsivity in the general population.

Validity of the diagnostic construct of ADHD across the lifespan was reviewed recently in the National Institute for Health and Clinical Excellence (NICE) guidelines [13] and summarized by Asherson and colleagues and the European Network Adult ADHD [11,14]. The criteria applied in the NICE guideline were based on the Washington University Diagnostic Criteria, which have been widely used and are similar to the approaches taken to define disorders for the DSM and the International Classification of Diseases (ICD). Additional evidence to support validity comes from the characteristic response of ADHD symptoms to specific treatment interventions (reviewed in Chapters 7 and 8).

The main validating criteria for ADHD in adults are as follows [13]:

- the phenomena of hyperactivity, inattention, and impulsivity cluster together;
- ADHD symptoms are distinguishable from other traits;
- the phenomena of hyperactivity, inattention, and impulsivity are not distinguishable from the normal spectrum. They lie on a continuum and the disorder is defined by the number and severity of symptoms and their link to clinical and psychosocial impairments;
- the clusters of symptoms that define ADHD are associated with significant clinical and psychosocial impairments;
- there are characteristic patterns of developmental change associated with the symptoms that define ADHD;
- there is consistent evidence of genetic, environmental, and neurobiological factors associated with ADHD;
- there is a characteristic reduction of the symptoms of ADHD after treatment with specific medications (see Chapter 7).

Main validating criteria

Symptom clustering

ADHD symptoms are consistently found to cluster together in clinical and population samples. The majority of studies support a two-factor model, with a single factor covering hyperactivity and impulsivity and a separate one for inattention. This factor structure may change with age as some adult studies suggest three separate factors for hyperactivity, impulsivity and inattention. Latent class analyses cluster symptoms into groups that are similar but not identical to DSM-IV subtypes [15].

More recent studies that have compared a range of different factor models support a hierarchical model with a general factor and two specific factors, one for the hyperactivity-impulsivity domain and one for inattention (Figure 3.2) [16,17].

Distinguishing symptoms

One of the main distinctions addressed in the literature is between ADHD and conduct problems. In childhood, the majority of studies find separate

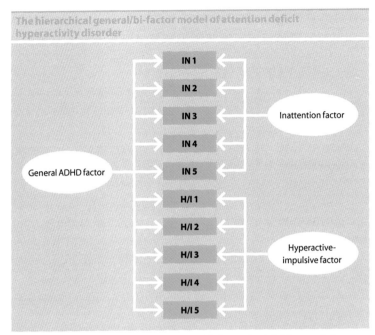

Figure 3.2 The hierarchical general/bi-factor model of attention deficit hyperactivity disorder. This model provides a better fit than the alternative model of two correlated dimensions of inattentive (IN) and hyperactive-impulsive (H/I) symptoms, indicating that ADHD represents a general factor combining both IN and H/I symptoms, in addition to two separate factors. This model fits well with the DSM-IV conceptualization of the three clinical subtypes of ADHD (predominantly inattentive subtype; predominantly hyperactive-impulsive subtype; combined subtype). ADHD, attention deficit hyperactivity disorder; DSM, Diagnostic and Statistical Manual of Mental Disorders. Adapted from Toplak et al [16,17].

but correlated factors for oppositional behavior and conduct problems. Although some studies have not been able to separate oppositional behavior from the hyperactive-impulsive symptom domain, there is consistent separation between oppositionality and inattention [18].

Available data indicate that whilst ADHD often precedes the development of conduct problems, the reverse does not occur [19]. Twin studies have found overlapping genetic influences between ADHD and conduct problems during childhood, but also suggest that there are shared environmental risks that appear to mediate the risk for conduct problems, but not ADHD [20]. These data suggest that ADHD in childhood acts as a risk factor for the development of conduct problems and that the development of conduct problems in the context of ADHD is likely to be mediated by both genetic and environmental factors.

An interesting, more specific, observation is that a particular genotype of the *catechol-O-methyl transferase (COMT)* gene that leads to increased breakdown of dopamine is associated with the development of antisocial behavior in children and adolescents with ADHD, a finding that has been reported in four separate samples (Figure 3.3) [21,22].

In general, high rates of comorbid conditions are known to co-occur in adults with ADHD, including autism spectrum disorder (ASD), specific reading difficulties, and motor coordination disorders. While these disorders are represented by symptom clusters that are distinct from ADHD in clinical and population samples, the evidence from family and twin studies is that their association with ADHD can be explained by shared genetic risk factors [23]. These most likely represent the so-called pleiotropic effects of genes by which common sets of overlapping genes lead to multiple different neurobiological and neurodevelopmental outcomes.

The distinction between ADHD in adults and commonly co-occurring symptoms, syndromes, and disorders is discussed in Chapter 6.

Distinguishing ADHD from the normal range of hyperactivity, inattention, and impulsivity

ADHD symptoms are continuously distributed throughout the general population in both children and adults. Furthermore, there is no distinct threshold that separates ADHD from the normal range of behavior [24]. In this sense, ADHD is comparable to other disorders that represent the extremes of normally occurring traits, such as hypertension, obesity, anxiety, and depression. For these conditions, the clinical disorder can be distinguished from the normal range in four main ways:

- severity (extreme nature) of symptoms compared to population norms;
- temporal persistence of symptoms from childhood to adulthood;
- association with significant levels of functional impairment during childhood, adolescence, and adulthood;
- risk for the development of co-occurring disorders.

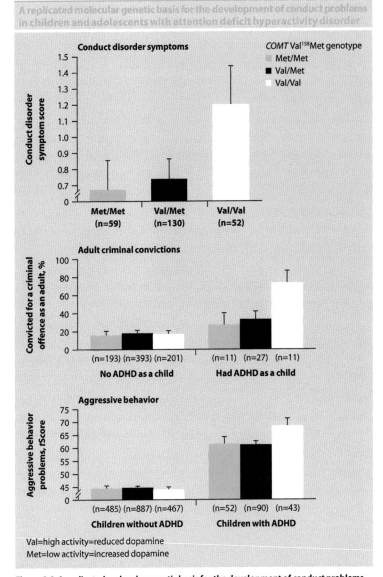

Figure 3.3 A replicated molecular genetic basis for the development of conduct problems in children and adolescents with attention deficit hyperactivity disorder. The first study is a sample of children with ADHD. The other two studies are longitudinal population samples which show that the *COMT* gene is only a risk factor for the development of later antisocial behavior in the groups that had ADHD as children. ADHD, attention deficit hyperactivity disorder; COMT, catechol-O-methyl transferase. Adapted from Caspi et al [21].

Association of ADHD with clinical and psychosocial impairments

A wide range of impairments are associated with ADHD in adults. These range from subjective impairments, such as distress from ADHD symptoms and low self esteem, to more objective impairments such as relationship problems, poor work performance, and increased accident rates [25–28]. Adults with ADHD also suffer from increased rates of academic difficulties, troubled family relationships, social difficulties, and conduct problems [25–28]. Increased rates of antisocial behavior, drug addiciton, and mood and anxiety disorders have been demonstrated in both cross-sectional and longitudinal follow-up studies [28,29]. Patients with ADHD also have increased rates of unemployment, poor work performance, lower educational performance, and a higher number of traffic violations, accidents, and criminal convictions [3,14,25–29].

Association of attention deficit hyperactivity disorder with genetic, environmental, and neurobiological factors

ADHD is associated with a wide range of genetic [23], environmental [30], and neurobiological [31–34] measures. Both genetic and environmental factors are likely to play an important role in the etiology of ADHD. However, unraveling the causal processes involved in ADHD has proved very difficult because many of the environmental and neurobiological variables that are associated with ADHD represent correlated rather than direct causal factors. One example of this is maternal smoking during pregnancy, which has consistently been shown to be associated with increased rates of ADHD among offspring. However, recent evidence has shown that this association reflects genetic risks that are shared between the mother and their offspring, rather than a direct toxic effect of exposure to smoking on the developing fetus [35].

Etiology

ADHD is a heterogeneous condition with multiple etiological factors involved in the risk for developing the clinical syndrome [36,37]. Family and twin studies demonstrate the importance of genetic factors, while cognitive and neuroimaging studies identify neurobiological processes associated with ADHD, some of which may mediate the genetic and environmental risks.

There is an ongoing debate about the relative importance of different cortical and subcortical brain regions, and the primary cognitive and neurobiological processes involved. It now seems likely that interactions between two or more key processes are critical to both the development and persistence of ADHD across the lifespan. Environmental risks include early and severe deprivation and exposure to prenatal risk factors such as maternal stress during pregnancy, low birth weight and premature birth [30,38].

Family and genetic studies

Family studies show that ADHD tends to aggregate in families, with a 5- to 10-fold increase in rates of ADHD among first-degree relatives of ADHD probands [24,39]. Numerous twin studies show that the familial aggregation of ADHD results from genetic factors, with correlations for ADHD symptoms among identical (monozygotic) twins being approximately twice those among nonidentical (dizygotic) twins, with an average heritability across studies of 70–80% [9,40].

Most twin studies indicate a limited role for shared environmental factors [40]. However, the environment is still likely to play an important role in three main ways:

- there may be unique environmental effects on individuals that explain differences between siblings and other close relatives;
- environmental factors may interact with genetic factors;
- heritability may be high in ADHD because the environmental risks are highly ubiquitous (ie, showing little variation in exposure).

Heritability of attention deficit hyperactivity disorder in adults

Family studies have found a particularly high familial risk among the siblings and parents of children with ADHD that persists into adolescence, and high rates of ADHD have also been reported among the offspring of parents with ADHD [39]. These findings suggest that ADHD that persists into adulthood may give risk to higher familial risks than ADHD that shows recovery during adolescence. This conclusion has not received strong support from twin studies of ADHD symptoms, which in adults have shown lower heritability estimates (around 30–40%) than those reported for childhood ADHD [41]. However, recent data from a UK twin sample found that this could result from rater effects, because in young adolescents, parent and teacher ratings give rise to higher heritability estimates than self ratings. In a large Swedish sample of young adult twins, when parent report and self-report data in adults were combined, the heritability of ADHD was found to be around 80%, which is very similar to that seen in children (Figure 3.4) [42].

Molecular genetic studies

The high heritability of ADHD symptoms during childhood and adolescence has led to international efforts to identify genetic variation that increases risk for the disorder [43] (Figure 3.5). Initial studies focused on candidate genes, particularly genes involved in the function and regulation of dopamine and other neurotransmitter systems involved in the response to treatment with stimulants. These studies identified several genes as being associated with ADHD, with the most consistent evidence for the dopamine D4 and D5 receptor genes [43]. Other candidate genes have been implicated, although further studies are required to confirm or refute these findings [44].

Several genome-wide association studies of ADHD have now been completed [45]. These studies have identified certain neurodevelopmental

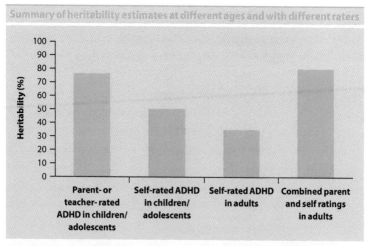

Figure 3.4 Summary of heritability estimates at different ages and with different raters.
ADHD, attention deficit hyperactivity disorder. Adapted from Asherson [23].

genes, such as cadherin 13, which is thought to have a role in neuronal migration and development, although evidence is not yet incontrovertible. Approaches that investigate groups of functionally related genes have been more successful in identifying sets of genes involved in neurite outgrowth and other basic neuronal processes (Figure 3.5) [46].

Rare copy number variants (CNVs) are also associated with ADHD. CNVs are submicroscopic deletions or duplications of chromosomal segments. In ADHD there is an approximately twofold increase in the number of CNVs compared to controls, particularly duplications that span functional gene regions [47,48]. CNVs seen in ADHD cases overlap with those identified in two other neurodevelopmental disorders: autism and schizophrenia. The finding that rare copy number variants of some genes increases risk across several psychiatric and neurodevelopmental disorders is a key finding that has emerged from genome-wide association studies and may provide a partial explanation for high rates of observed comorbidity.

Environmental risks

Several environmental measures have been identified that are associated with ADHD. These studies are almost entirely completed in childhood, so there is limited information on environmental risks associated with persistence of the disorder in adult life. Furthermore, even where associations with environmental measures are identified, it is difficult to separate out the direct 'toxic' effects of environmental exposures from genetic risks.

A review of all potential environmental risks for ADHD identified the following environmental exposures as being associated with ADHD [30]:

- **Diet:** diet appears to be a factor that can increase levels of ADHD symptoms in some cases [49,50]. However, there is as yet limited evidence that dietary control provides effective treatment for ADHD in most cases.
- **Exposure to toxins:** exposure to lead and mercury is associated with an increase in levels of ADHD symptoms [51].
- **Pregnancy and delivery complications:** adverse events during pregnancy may increase risk of ADHD in some cases. The best evidence of a link to early developmental problems is the association with low birth weight and prematurity [52].

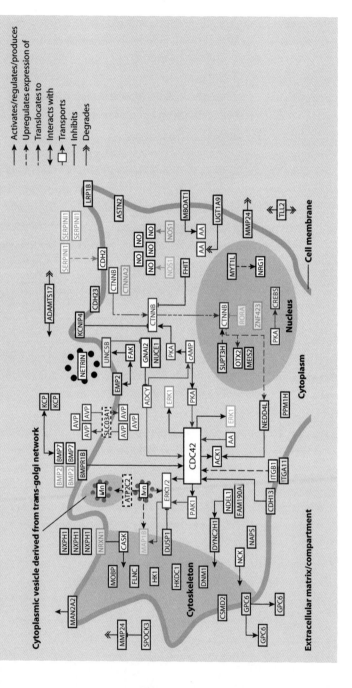

Illustration of the ADHD neurodevelopmental signalling pathways for directed neurite outgrowth

- **Fetal alcohol exposure:** several studies show associations between fetal alcohol exposure and ADHD symptoms [53–55].

- **Maternal smoking during pregnancy:** maternal smoking has been widely reported to be associated with ADHD, yet recent studies indicate that this is unlikely to be a direct toxic effect, as no environmental risk is seen once genetic factors are controlled for [34].

- **Psychosocial adversity:** low economic status and severe maltreatment may be associated with ADHD. Rutter and colleagues found high rates of inattention and overactivity in Romanian adoptees that were exposed to severe early deprivation [56]. Interestingly, the main risks appeared to occur with exposure to the deprived environments that went from 6 months of life onward, with no apparent risk if exposure was stopped before 6 months. Biederman identified psychosocial adversity and comorbidity as predictors of persistence of ADHD into adult life [57].

Figure 3.5 Illustration of the ADHD neurodevelopmental signalling pathways for directed neurite outgrowth (see opposite). The genes in yellow were identified from analysis of five genome-wide association studies for ADHD. The genes in green have reported rare copy number variants in ADHD. The genes in red show altered expression in response to stimulant medications. ACK1, activated Cdc42-associated kinase 1; ADAMTS17, a disintegrin and metalloproteinase with thrombospondin motifs metallopeptidase with thrombospondin type 1 motif, 17; ADCY, adenylyl cyclase; AVP, arginine vasopressin; BMP, bone morphogenetic protein; cAMP, cyclic adenosine monophosphate; CDC42, cell division control protein 42 homolog; CDH13, cadherin 13, H-cadherin (heart); CDH2, cadherin-2; CDH23, cadherin-related 23; CREBS, cAMP response element binding proteins; CSMD2, CUB and sushi multiple domains 2; CTNNA/B, catenin cadherin-associated protein; DNM1, dynamin 1; DUSP1, dual-specificity protein phosphatase 1; DYNC2H1, dynein, cytoplasmic 2, heavy chain 1; EMP, epithelial membrane protein; ERK1/2, extracellular signal-regulated kinase 1/2; FAM190A, family with sequence similarity 190, member A; FHIT, fragile histidine triad protein; GPC6, glypican 6; HK1, hexokinase-1; HKDC1, hexokinase domain containing 1; ITGA11, integrin α-11; ITGB1, integrin beta-1; KCNIP4, kv channel interacting protein 4; KCP, kielin/chordin-like protein; LRP1B, low-density lipoprotein receptor-related protein 1B; MAN2A2, mannosidase, α, class 2A, member 2; MBOAT1, membrane-bound O-acyltransferase domain containing 1; MEIS2, meis homeobox 2; MMP24, matrix metallopeptidase 24; Mn, manganese; MYT1L, myelin transcription factor 1-like; NAPS, nucleoid-associated proteins; NCK, noncatalytic region of tyrosine kinase adaptor protein; NDEL1, nuclear distribution gene E homolog-like 1; NEDD4L, neural precursor cell expressed, developmentally down-regulated 4-like; NO, nitric oxide; NOS1, nitric oxide synthase 1; NRG1, neurogulin 1; NRXN1, neurexin-1-α; NXPH1, neurexophilin-1; OTX2, orthodenticle homeobox 2; PAK1, p21 protein-activated kinase 1; PKA, protein kinase A; PPM1H, protein phosphatase, Mg2+/Mn2+ dependent, 1H; RORA, retinoic acid-related orphan receptor α; SERPIN1, serine protease inhibitor 1; SLCO3A1, solute carrier organic anion transporter family, member 3A; SPOCK3, sparc/osteonectin, cwcv and kazal-like domains proteoglycan (testican) 3; SUPT3H, suppressor of Ty 3 homolog; TLL2, tolloid-like 2; UGT1A9, UDP glucuronosyltransferase 1 family, polypeptide A9; UNC5B, unc-5 homolog B; ZNF423, zinc finger protein 423. Adapted from Poelmans et al [46].

Cognitive processes

A wide range of cognitive performance deficits have been identified in ADHD groups compared to controls, and similar deficits are seen in both children and adults with ADHD [58,59]. The cognitive deficits relate to several distinct processes, and both cortical and subcortical regions and their connections have been implicated. Some of the most prominent neuropsychological models of ADHD are listed in Table 3.2.

There is considerable debate about whether the multiple cognitive performance deficits observed in ADHD result from one or two key underlying processes or whether they indicate a more extensive heterogeneity in the neurobiological processes that give rise to the symptoms and behaviors that characterize ADHD. Heterogeneity could take the form of multiple interacting processes, or could lead to 'neurobiological' subtypes with different outcomes and response to treatments. The association of particular cognitive performance measures with ADHD does not in itself imply a mediating causal process as the cognitive impairments might reflect the multiple outcomes of genetic and environmental risks. Furthermore, many of the cognitive deficits are not specific to ADHD and are seen in other mental health conditions. Based on current data, many uncertainties remain about the nature of the processes that underlie ADHD, although cognitive deficits are consistently found to be associated with the disorder and may be linked to functional impairments (Figure 3.6).

Neuroimaging and electrophysiology

Structural changes

In children with ADHD, smaller volumes are seen in the frontal lobes, basal ganglia, cerebellum, and parietotemporal regions. Studies in adults have reported reduced volumes in similar brain regions. More specifically, decreased volume in left orbitofrontal cortex, and decreased overall volume of cortical gray matter, right anterior cingulate and left superior/dorsolateral prefrontal cortex has been observed. In addition, increased volume of the nucleus accumbens and the size of white matter tracts connecting the anterior cingulate with the dorsolateral prefrontal cortex has been noted [33]. Overall, studies show similar structural deficits in children and adults with ADHD in prefrontal, cingulate, and parietotemporal brain regions.

Prominent cognitive models of attention deficit hyperactivity disorder

Executive dysfunction	Deficits in higher order cognitive processes, such as planning, sequencing, reasoning, holding attention to a task, working memory, and inhibition of inappropriate and selection of appropriate behaviors. Inhibition has been proposed as one of the key deficits in adults with ADHD, although earlier sensory deficits are found to precede motor inhibitory responses [60].
State regulation	Nonoptimal energetic state can explain performance deficits in ADHD. Performance efficiency is considered to be the product of elementary cognitive stages and their energy distribution. The elementary stages include stimulus encoding, memory search, binary decision, and motor preparation. The availability of these basic processes is related to arousal and activation levels of individuals. Effort is needed to meet task demands and compensate for suboptimal arousal or activation states [61].
Delay aversion	Delay aversion accounts for the observation that individuals with ADHD do not like to wait. It is a motivational account of ADHD, in contrast to more cognitive explanations. Inattentiveness and hyperactivity are proposed to result from attempts to reduce subjective experience of delay in situations where delay cannot be avoided [62].
Dual pathway models	1. The first dual pathway hypothesis proposed the existence of two distinct pathways to ADHD: delay aversion reflecting motivational factors, and inhibitory deficits reflecting poor cortical or executive control [63]. 2. Multivariate family and twin analyses identified two familial cognitive factors that account for most of the familial effects on ADHD: the first factor indexed by reaction time and reaction time variability, the second factor indexed by omission and commission errors. These measures are proposed to reflect state-regulation and executive function deficits, respectively [64]. 3. The identification of two key pathways in the multivariate family and twin studies is reflected in a developmental model proposed by Halperin that suggests that an early enduring primary neurodevelopmental abnormality leads to impairments that are modified as executive functions mature throughout development. It is proposed that the balance between these two processes leads to individual differences in persistence of ADHD during adolescence and early adulthood [65].
Dynamic developmental theory	The theory suggests that there are two main behavioral mechanisms underpinning the symptoms of ADHD: altered reinforcement of novel behavior and deficient extinction of inadequate behavior. The basis for the theory lies in the delay-of-reinforcement gradient between response to a stimulus and reinforcement of that response. It is proposed that in ADHD, the 'window of opportunity' for reinforcement is smaller, so that socially desirable behaviors are not reinforced fast enough, leading to symptoms associated with ADHD [66].
Default mode network	Attentional lapses often seen during task performance in ADHD could indicate a role of DMN interference. The default DMN represents brain regions that are found to be activated during resting conditions. During normal task performance the DMN is attenuated. However, in ADHD, inefficient and variable performance may arise because during goal-directed tasks, some patients with ADHD may not effectively attenuate the activity of the DMN. This may cause the DMN activity to intrude on task performance and thus cause periodic lapses of attention [67].

Table 3.2 Prominent cognitive models of attention deficit hyperactivity disorder. DMN, default mode network. Adapted from Johnson et al [37].

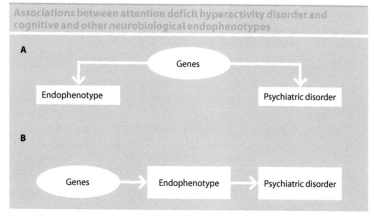

Figure 3.6 A and B Associations between attention deficit hyperactivity disorder and cognitive and other neurobiological endophenotypes. Genes that confer risk for ADHD do not necessarily indicate causal pathways from genetic risks to the clinical disorder. Many of the associated impairments will reflect pleiotropic processes that have no direct causal role (A). Others may mediate genetic effects on behavior. (B) In clinical practice, both types of impairments are important because they reflect cognitive/neurobiological deficits that are seen in people with ADHD. RVEP, residual variance endophenotype. Adapted with permission from Kendler and Neale [68].

Maturational delay hypothesis

A longitudinal study suggested that in ADHD there is a delay in the age at which peak cortical thickness is reached [69]. This is thought to indicate a maturational lag of brain myelination in ADHD compared to controls, although this does not imply 'catching up' during adulthood since both structural and functional impairments remain in adults with ADHD.

Functional imaging

Most neuroimaging research has been conducted in children with ADHD, although there are a growing number of studies on adults. A critical review of the data for ADHD found the following functional changes [70]:

- dysfunction in the frontal lobes during tasks that tap response inhibition, although there are some inconsistencies regarding the exact nature of the problem;
- dysfunction of temporal and parietal regions also play a part, mostly during tasks that tap attentional processes;
- consistent evidence shows that patients with ADHD demonstrate reduced activation of the striatum.

Default mode network studies

Evidence from studies examining spontaneous brain activity in youths with ADHD is consistent with a dysfunction in more general processes, rather than deficits pertaining to specific cognitive processes. Adults with ADHD have shown decreased functional connectivity between default mode network regions, which was also shown to relate to levels of ADHD symptoms [71].

Atypical prefrontal connectivity

Diffusion tensor imaging studies have further added to the structural findings in ADHD, by suggesting that ADHD is significantly associated with structural connectivity deficits in functionally relevant white matter tracts, especially in frontostriatal and certain corticocortical tracts [72]. Resting state functional imaging studies also implicate altered connectivity between the default mode network and frontostriatal networks (Figure 3.7).

Direct child versus adult attention deficit hyperactivity disorder studies

The question of whether the same functional impairments are seen in children and adults with ADHD is difficult to address based on currently available data, because studies have tended to use different cognitive task paradigms. Nevertheless, striking similarities have been identified in studies that have used the same paradigms affecting inferior frontal parietal, caudate and parietal regions [33]. A recent review and analysis of a drug-naive longitudinal sample from childhood to adulthood suggest that ADHD is associated with brain abnormalities in fronto-cortical and fronto-subcortical systems that mediate the control of cognition and motivation [32].

Electrophysiological investigations

Electroencephalogram studies

The most consistent finding from electroencephalogram measures is of increased theta activity in adults with ADHD compared with controls. Nevertheless, not all studies have been able to replicate these findings

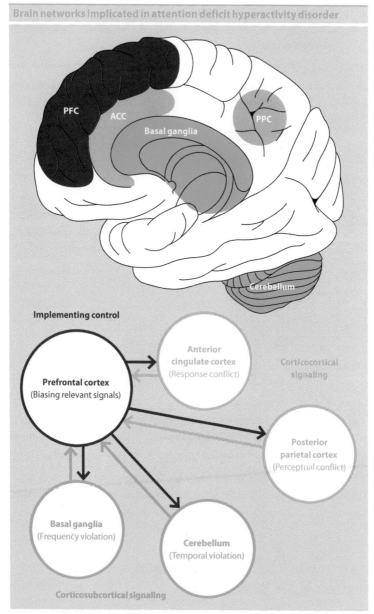

Figure 3.7 Brain networks implicated in attention deficit hyperactivity disorder. ACC, anterior cingulate cortex; PFC, prefrontal cortex; PPC, posterior parietal cortex. Adapted with permission from Liston et al [72].

and further work is needed to clarify the robustness of this association in clinical samples of ADHD [34].

Event-related potential studies

Event-related potential studies have been successful in identifying consistent findings in children and adults with ADHD for early components of attention. In particular, using a cued continuous performance task, similar findings were reported in children and adults with ADHD. These findings suggested that response inhibition is unlikely to reflect a primary deficit in ADHD, because in this task inhibitory response deficits are preceded by deficits in early preparatory processing [73,74].

Molecular imaging

In the last decade, a series of single-photon emission computed tomography (SPECT) and positron emission tomography (PET) studies investigated the dopamine system in adults with ADHD as compared to healthy controls. Most studies have relatively small samples sizes, and some findings are controversial [75]. For example, one of the most ambitious PET studies ever performed in a psychiatric population was carried out by Volkow et al [76,77], in which never-medicated adult ADHD patients (n=55) and healthy controls (n=44) were scanned with [^{11}C]raclopride and [^{11}C]cocaine. ADHD patients showed significantly lower availability of D2/D3 dopamine receptors and reduced density of the dopamine transporter (DAT). Furthermore, the severity of ADHD symptoms and motivational deficits correlated with striatal dopamine receptor density. An important confounding factor in these studies is previous exposure to stimulant medication. A meta-analysis of DAT studies found an impact of previous medication on striatal DAT availability [78]: never-medicated patients had reduced DAT, whereas previous medication seems to normalize or increase DAT availability. Other neurotransmitter systems have yet to be studied with molecular imaging methods in ADHD.

Overall, we can conclude that ADHD appears to involve multiple brain systems and that brain abnormalities associated with ADHD persist throughout the lifespan.

References

1   Polanczyk G, de Lima MS, Horta BL, et al. The worldwide prevalence of ADHD: a systematic review and metaregression analysis. *Am J Psychiatry*. 2007;164:942-948.

2   Ford T, Goodman R, Meltzer H. The British Child and Adolescent Mental Health Survey 1999: the prevalence of DSM-IV disorders. *J Am Acad Child Adolesc Psychiatry*. 2003;42:1203-1211.

3   Fayyad J, De Graaf R, Kessler R, et al. Cross-national prevalence and correlates of adult attention-deficit hyperactivity disorder. *Br J Psychiatry*. 2007;190:402-409.

4   Kessler RC, Adler L, Berkley R, et al. The prevalence and correlates of adult ADHD in the United States: results from the National Comorbidity Survey Replication. *Am J Psychiatry*. 2006;163:716-723.

5   Simon V, Czobor P, Balint S, et al. Prevalence and correlates of adult attention-deficit hyperactivity disorder: meta-analysis. *Br J Psychiatry*. 2009;194:204-211.

6   Faraone SV, Biederman J, Mick E. The age-dependent decline of attention deficit hyperactivity disorder: a meta-analysis of follow-up studies. *Psychol Med*. 2006;36:159-165.

7   McCarthy S, Asherson P, Coghill D, et al. Attention-deficit hyperactivity disorder: treatment discontinuation in adolescents and young adults. *Br J Psychiatry*. 2009;194:273-277.

8   McArdle P, Prosser J, Kolvin I. Prevalence of psychiatric disorder: with and without psychosocial impairment. *Eur Child Adolesc Psychiatry*. 2004:13:347-353.

9   Faraone SV, Biederman J. What is the prevalence of adult ADHD? Results of a population screen of 966 adults. *J Atten Disord*. 2005;9:384-391.

10 Kooij JJ, Buitelaar JK, van den Oord EJ, et al. Internal and external validity of attention-deficit hyperactivity disorder in a population-based sample of adults. *Psychol Med*. 2005;35:817-827.

11 Asherson P, Adamou M, Bolea B, et al. Is ADHD a valid diagnosis in adults? Yes. *BMJ*. 2010;340:c549.

12 Moncrieff J, Timimi S. Is ADHD a valid diagnosis in adults? No. *BMJ*. 2010;340:c547.

13 National Institute for Health and Clinical Excellent (NICE). Attention deficit hyperactivity disorder clinical guidelines 72: attention deficit hyperactivity disorder: diagnosis and management of ADHD in children, young people and adults. NICE website. www.nice.org.uk/CG72. Accessed August 25, 2012.

14 Kooij SJ, Bejerot S, Blackwell A, et al. European consensus statement on diagnosis and treatment of adult ADHD: The European Network Adult ADHD. *BMC Psychiatry*. 2010;10:67.

15 Todd RD, Rasmussen ER, Neuman RJ, et al. Familiality and heritability of subtypes of attention deficit hyperactivity disorder in a population sample of adolescent female twins. *Am J Psychiatry*. 2001;158:1891-1898.

16 Toplak ME, Pitch A, Flora DB, et al. The unity and diversity of inattention and hyperactivity/impulsivity in ADHD: evidence for a general factor with separable dimensions. *J Abnorm Child Psychol*. 2009;37:1137-1150.

17 Toplak ME, Sorge GB, Flora DB, et al. The hierarchical factor model of ADHD: Invariant across age and national groupings? *J Child Psychol Psychiatry*. 2011;53:292-303.

18 Wood AC, Rijsdijk F, Asherson P, et al. Hyperactive-impulsive symptom scores and oppositional behaviors reflect alternate manifestations of a single liability. *Behav Genet*. 2009;39:447-460.

19 Taylor E, Chadwick O, Heptinstall E, et al. Hyperactivity and conduct problems as risk factors for adolescent development. *J Am Acad Child Adolesc Psychiatry*. 1996;35:1213-1226.

20 Thapar A, Harrington R, McGuffin P. Examining the comorbidity of ADHD-related behaviors and conduct problems using a twin study design. *Br J Psychiatry*. 2001;179:224-229.

21 Caspi A, Langley K, Milne B, et al. A replicated molecular genetic basis for subtyping antisocial behavior in children with attention-deficit/hyperactivity disorder. *Arch Gen Psychiatry*. 2008;65:203-210.

22 Langley K, Heron J, O'Donovan MC, et al. Genotype link with extreme antisocial behavior: the contribution of cognitive pathways. *Arch Gen Psychiatry*. 2010;67:1317-1323.

23 Asherson P, Gurling H. Quantitative and molecular genetics of ADHD. *Curr Top Behav Neurosci.* Curr Top Behav Neurosci. 2012;9:239-272.

24 Chen W, Zhou K, Sham P, et al. DSM-IV combined type ADHD shows familial association with sibling trait scores: a sampling strategy for QTL linkage. *Am J Med Genet B Neuropsychiatr Genet.* 2008;147B:1450-1460.

25 Barkley RA, Murphy KR, Dupaul GI, et al. Driving in young adults with attention deficit hyperactivity disorder: knowledge, performance, adverse outcomes, and the role of executive functioning. *J Int Neuropsychol Soc.* 2002;8:655-672.

26 de Graaf R, Kessler RC, Fayyad J, et al. The prevalence and effects of adult attention-deficit/ hyperactivity disorder (ADHD) on the performance of workers: results from the WHO World Mental Health Survey Initiative. *Occup Environ Med.* 2008;65:835-842.

27 Gau SS, Kessler RC, Tseng WL, et al. Association between sleep problems and symptoms of attention-deficit/hyperactivity disorder in young adults. *Sleep.* 2007;30:195-201.

28 Kessler RC, Adler L, Ames M, et al. The prevalence and effects of adult attention deficit/ hyperactivity disorder on work performance in a nationally representative sample of workers. *J Occup Environ Med.* 2005;47:565-572.

29 Kooij JJS, Aeckerlin LP, Buitelaar JK. Functioning, comorbidity and treatment of 141 adults with attention deficit hyperactivity disorder (ADHD) at a Psychiatric Outpatients' Department. [Dutch]. *Ned Tijdschr Geneeskd.* 2001;145:1498-1501.

30 Banerjee TD, Middleton F, Faraone SV. Environmental risk factors for attention-deficit hyperactivity disorder. *Acta Paediatr.* 2007;96:1269-1274.

31 Castellanos FX, Tannock, R. Neuroscience of attention-deficit/hyperactivity disorder: the search for endophenotypes. *Nat Rev Neurosci.* 2002;3:617-628.

32 Cubillo A, Halari R, Smith A, et al. A review of fronto-striatal and fronto-cortical brain abnormalities in children and adults with Attention Deficit Hyperactivity Disorder (ADHD) and new evidence for dysfunction in adults with ADHD during motivation and attention. *Cortex.* 2011;48:194-215.

33 Cubillo A, Rubia K. Structural and functional brain imaging in adult attention-deficit/ hyperactivity disorder. *Expert Rev Neurother.* 2010;10:603-620.

34 Tye C, McLoughlin G, Kuntsi J, et al. Electrophysiological markers of genetic risk for attention deficit hyperactivity disorder. *Expert Rev Mol Med.* 2011;13:e9.

35 Thapar A, Rice F, Hay D, et al. Prenatal smoking might not cause attention-deficit/hyperactivity disorder: evidence from a novel design. *Biol Psychiatry.* 2009;66:722-727.

36 Coghill D, Nigg J, Rothenberger A, et al. Whither causal models in the neuroscience of ADHD? *Dev Sci.* 2005;8:105-114.

37 Johnson KA, Wiersema JR, Kuntsi J. What would Karl Popper say? Are current psychological theories of ADHD falsifiable? *Behav Brain Funct.* 2009;5:15.

38 Stevens SE, Sonuga-Barke EJ, Kreppner JM, et al. Inattention/overactivity following early severe institutional deprivation: presentation and associations in early adolescence. *J Abnorm Child Psychol.* 2008;36:385-398.

39 Faraone SV, Biederman J, Monuteaux MC. Toward guidelines for pedigree selection in genetic studies of attention deficit hyperactivity disorder. *Genet Epidemiol.* 2000;18:1-16.

40 Burt SA. Rethinking environmental contributions to child and adolescent psychopathology: a meta-analysis of shared environmental influences. *Psychol Bull.* 2009;135:608-637.

41 Boomsma DI, Saviouk V, Hottenga JJ, et al. Genetic epidemiology of attention deficit hyperactivity disorder (ADHD index) in adults. *PLoS One.* 2010;5:e10621.

42 Freitag CM, Rohde LA, Lempp T, Romanos M. Phenotypic and measurement influences on heritability estimates in childhood ADHD. *Eur Child Adolesc Psychiatry.* 2010;19:311-323.

43 Li D, Sham PC, Owen MJ, et al. Meta-analysis shows significant association between dopamine system genes and attention deficit hyperactivity disorder (ADHD). *Hum Mol Genet.* 2006;15:2276-2284.

44 Gizer IR, Ficks C, Waldman ID. Candidate gene studies of ADHD: a meta-analytic review. *Hum Genet*. 2009;126:51-90.

45 Franke B, Neale BM, Faraone SV. Genome-wide association studies in ADHD. *Hum Genet*. 2009;126:13-50.

46 Poelmans G, Pauls DL, Buitelaar JK, et al. Integrated genome-wide association study findings: identification of a neurodevelopmental network for attention deficit hyperactivity disorder. *Am J Psychiatry*. 2011;168:365-377.

47 Williams NM, Franke B, Mick E, et al. Genome-wide analysis of copy number variants in attention deficit hyperactivity disorder: the role of rare variants and duplications at 15q13.3. *Am J Psychiatry*. 2011;169:195-204.

48 Williams NM, Zaharieva I, Martin A, et al. Rare chromosomal deletions and duplications in attention-deficit hyperactivity disorder: a genome-wide analysis. *Lancet*. 2010;376:1401-1408.

49 Pelsser LM, Frankena K, Toorman J, et al. Effects of a restricted elimination diet on the behavior of children with attention-deficit hyperactivity disorder (INCA study): a randomised controlled trial. *Lancet*. 2011;377:494-503.

50 Stevenson J, Sonuga-Barke E, McCann D, et al The role of histamine degradation gene polymorphisms in moderating the effects of food additives on children's ADHD symptoms. *Am J Psychiatry*. 2010;167:1108-1111.

51 Nigg JT, Nikolas M, Mark Knottnerus G., et al. Confirmation and extension of association of blood lead with attention-deficit/hyperactivity disorder (ADHD) and ADHD symptom domains at population-typical exposure levels. *J Child Psychol Psychiatry*. 2010;51:58-65.

52 Aylward GP. Neurodevelopmental outcomes of infants born prematurely. *J Dev Behav Pediatr*. 2005;26:427-440.

53 Oesterheld JR, Wilson A. ADHD and FAS (Letter to the editor). *J Am Acad Child Adolesc Psychiatry*. 1997;36:1163.

54 Steinhausen HC, Willms J, Spohr HL. Long-term psychopathological and cognitive outcome of children with fetal alcohol syndrome. *J Am Acad Child Adolesc Psychiatry*. 1993;32:990-994.

55 Streissguth AP, Bookstein FL, Sampson PD, Barr HM. Attention: Prenatal alcohol and continuities of vigilance and attentional problems from 4 through 14 years. *Dev Psychopathol*. 1995;7:419-446.

56 Rutter M, Colvert E, Kreppner J, et al. Early adolescent outcomes for institutionally-deprived and non-deprived adoptees. I: disinhibited attachment. *J Child Psychol Psychiatry*. 2007;48:17-30.

57 Biederman J, Petty CR, Clarke A, et al. Predictors of persistent ADHD: An 11-year follow-up study. *J Psychiatr Res*. 2010;45:150-155.

58 Boonstra AM, Oosterlaan J, Sergeant JA, et al. Executive functioning in adult ADHD: a meta-analytic review. *Psychol Med*. 2005;35:1097-1108.

59 Hervey AS, Epstein JN, Curry JF. Neuropsychology of adults with attention-deficit/hyperactivity disorder: a meta-analytic review. *Neuropsychology*. 2004;18:485-503.

60 Barkley RA. Behavioral inhibition, sustained attention, and executive functions: constructing a unifying theory of ADHD. *Psychol Bull*. 1997;121:65-94.

61 Sergeant JA. Modeling attention-deficit/hyperactivity disorder: a critical appraisal of the cognitive-energetic model. *Biol Psychiatry*. 2005;57:1248-1255.

62 Marco R, Miranda A, Schlotz W, et al. Delay and reward choice in ADHD: an experimental test of the role of delay aversion. *Neuropsychology*. 2009;23:367-380.

63 Sonuga-Barke EJ. The dual pathway model of AD/HD: an elaboration of neuro-developmental characteristics. *Neurosci Biobehav Rev*. 2003;27:593-604.

64 Kuntsi J, Wood AC, Rijsdijk F, et al. Separation of cognitive impairments in attention-deficit/hyperactivity disorder into 2 familial factors. *Arch Gen Psychiatry*. 2010:67:1159-1167.

65 Halperin JM, Trampush JW, Miller CJ, et al. Neuropsychological outcome in adolescents/young adults with childhood ADHD: profiles of persisters, remitters and controls. *J Child Psychol Psychiatry*. 2008;49:958-966.

66 Sagvolden T, Johansen EB, Aase H, et al. A dynamic developmental theory of attention-deficit/ hyperactivity disorder (ADHD) predominantly hyperactive/impulsive and combined subtypes. *Behav Brain Sci*. 2005;28:397-419.

67 Broyd SJ, Demanuele C, Debener S, et al. Default-mode brain dysfunction in mental disorders: a systematic review. *Neurosci Biobehav Rev*. 2009;33:279-296.

68 Kendler KS, Neale MC. Endophenotype: a conceptual analysis. *Mol Psychiatry*. 2010;15:789-797.

69 Shaw P, Eckstrand K, Sharp W, et al. Attention-deficit/hyperactivity disorder is characterized by a delay in cortical maturation. *Proc Natl Acad Sci USA*. 2007;104:19649-19654.

70 Paloyelis Y, Mehta MA, Kuntsi J, et al. Functional MRI in ADHD: a systematic literature review. *Expert Rev Neurother*. 2007;7:1337-1356.

71 Castellanos FX, Margulies DS, Kelly C, et al. Cingulate-precuneus interactions: a new locus of dysfunction in adult attention-deficit/hyperactivity disorder. *Biol Psychiatry*. 2008;63:332-337.

72 Liston C, Malter Cohen M, Teslovich T, et al. Atypical prefrontal connectivity in attention-deficit/ hyperactivity disorder: pathway to disease or pathological end point? *Biol Psychiatry*. 2011;69:1168-1177.

73 Banaschewski T, Brandeis D, Heinrich H, et al. Questioning inhibitory control as the specific deficit of ADHD-evidence from brain electrical activity. *J Neural Transm*. 2004;111:841-864.

74 McLoughlin G, Albrecht B, Banaschewski T, et al. Electrophysiological evidence for abnormal preparatory states and inhibitory processing in adult ADHD. *Behav Brain Funct*. 2010;6:66.

75 Del Campo N, Muller U, Sahakian B. Neural and behavioral endophenotypes in ADHD. In, JW Dalley, CS Carter (eds), *Brain Imaging in Behavioral Neuroscience (Current Topics in Behavioral Neurosciences, CTBN Series)* New York, NY: Springer; 2012.

76 Volkow ND, Wang GJ, Kollins SH, et al. Evaluating dopamine reward pathway in ADHD: clinical implications. *JAMA*. 2009;302:1084-1091.

77 Volkow ND, Wang GJ, Newcorn JH, et al. Motivation deficit in ADHD is associated with dysfunction of the dopamine reward pathway. *Mol Psychiatry*. 2011;16:1147-1154.

78 Fusar-Poli P, Rubia K, Rossi G, et al. Striatal dopamine transporter alterations in ADHD: pathophysiology or adaptation to psychostimulants? A meta-analysis. *Am J Psychiatry*. 2012;169:264-272.

Diagnostic assessment of attention deficit hyperactivity disorder in adults

Attention deficit hyperactivity disorder (ADHD) is a clinical syndrome defined by the presence of impairing levels of hyperactive, inattentive, and impulsive symptoms. Although cognitive deficits are associated with ADHD, not all people with ADHD appear impaired on cognitive tests, and none of the cognitive tests associated with ADHD are specific to the disorder. Thus, cognitive tests should not be used to determine the presence of the disorder. The diagnosis is made in the same way as for other common psychiatric disorders: by careful evaluation of the mental state and a full psychiatric evaluation, including developmental history, functional impairments, and current and past psychiatric history.

Key principles

ADHD is often considered to be a particularly difficult diagnosis to establish in adults, yet there is a considerable consensus among experts about the nature of the core syndrome and how to diagnose the disorder [1]. Certain principles should guide clinicians as follows:

- The diagnosis of ADHD can be distinguished from other common psychiatric disorders of ADHD.
- Diagnosis is no more difficult to make than the evaluation of other common mental health disorders such as anxiety or depression.

UKAAN, *Handbook for Attention Deficit Hyperactivity Disorder in Adults*, DOI: 10.1007/978-1-908517-79-1_4, © Springer Healthcare 2013

- ADHD in adults is a symptomatic disorder, with characteristic descriptions by patients of mental states that reflect the psychopathology of the disorder. ADHD does not just reflect behavioral problems.
- The disorder in adults is commonly misdiagnosed for other common mental health disorders. However, this can usually be avoided by paying attention to the characteristic early onset and trait-like course of the symptoms and impairments that define the disorder.
- ADHD is treatable in most cases and it is important for the wellbeing of patients who present with untreated ADHD to diagnose and treat the disorder.

Diagnosing attention deficit hyperactivity disorder in adults

When evaluating the diagnosis of ADHD in adults there are several key points to consider:

- the DSM-IV criteria;
- diagnostic interviews;
- age-adjusted criteria for symptoms;
- ADHD symptoms are trait like;
- associated symptoms and functional impairments;
- cognitive testing;
- behavioral aspects of the patient's mental state during their clinical evaluation;
- obtaining accurate accounts of symptoms;
- compensatory mechanisms used by the patient.

Diagnostic and Statistical Manual of Mental Disorders criteria

ADHD is a clinical syndrome defined by the presence of high levels of inattentive, hyperactive, and impulsive symptoms. When making a diagnosis, most clinicians use the *Diagnostic and Statistical Manual of Mental Disorders (DSM-IV)* criteria because the International Classification of

Disease (ICD-10) hyperkinetic disorder defines a restricted subgroup of patients with severe combined type ADHD [1] and does not allow many common forms of comorbidity and broader clinical presentations of the disorder. It is envisaged that most clinicians will move to DSM-V and ICD-11 once the revisions are published in their final form.

Diagnostic interview

The diagnosis should be made following a detailed clinical interview to evaluate the presence of inattention, hyperactivity, and impulsivity when they are severe and impairing. The key elements are:

- current ADHD symptoms;
- common associated symptoms of ADHD that do not appear in the DSM-IV criteria;
- retrospective (occurring in child or adolescent) ADHD symptoms;
- impairments associated with ADHD symptoms;
- comorbid symptoms, syndromes, and disorders.

Age-adjusted criteria for symptoms

Symptoms of ADHD change with developmental age. In most cases, inattentive symptoms in particular become more prominent relative to hyperactive-impulsive symptoms with age. However, when properly age-adjusted expressions of ADHD symptoms are taken into account, persistence of impairing levels of all ADHD symptoms are often seen. Furthermore, when hyperactivity-impulsivity does persist it can be particularly impairing. Examples of adult expressions of ADHD symptoms for each of the DSM-IV items are listed in Chapter 2 and also provided as examples within the Diagnostic Interview for ADHD in Adults (DIVA) clinical diagnostic interview [2] (see Appendix G).

Attention deficit hyperactivity disorder symptoms are trait-like

ADHD symptoms in adults are chronic and trait-like. They start during childhood or early adolescence and follow a trait-like course. For this reason, they are more easily mistaken for symptoms of a personality disorder than an episodic adult-onset disorder. When evaluating ADHD, clinicians should expect to see symptoms that start during childhood and follow a persistent and nonfluctuating course.

Associated symptoms and functional impairments

There are a range of additional symptoms and impairments that are commonly seen in ADHD and form part of the core syndrome. These should be used to support the diagnosis and may be the key presenting complaint in some cases. Some examples of typical presentations of ADHD and associated symptoms are listed in Table 4.1.

Cognitive testing

Although ADHD is associated with a range of impairments of cognition and measures of brain function, these features are insufficiently sensitive or specific and should not be used to include or exclude the disorder in clinical practice. Rather, they should be used to provide additional information on the range of impairments in patients that meet the diagnostic criteria for ADHD.

Common clinical presentations in attention deficit hyperactivity disorder	
1. Disorganization	Does not plan ahead
2. Forgetfulness	Misses appointments, loses things
3. Procrastination	Starts projects but does not complete
4. Time management problems	Always late
5. Premature shifting of activities	Starts something but then is quickly distracted by something else
6. Impulsive decisions	Spending, taking on projects, travelling, jobs, or social plans
7. Mood lability	Irritable or labile moods and low tolerance of frustration
8. Low boredom threshold	Gets bored easily once the novelty of an activity has worn off
9. Low self esteem	Often associated with life-long functional impairments
10. Variable performance	Both under- and over-focused on tasks, or focuses only on immediately rewarding tasks
11. Criminal offences	Speeding, road traffic accidents, taking illegal drugs
12. Unstable jobs and relationships	Unable to keep a job or maintain long-term relationships

Table 4.1 Common clinical presentations in attention deficit hyperactivity disorder.

Behavioral aspects of mental state during clinical evaluation

ADHD symptoms such as restlessness and distractibility may not be reflected in behaviors during clinical interviews. The reason for this is the sensitivity of the symptoms to stimulating or salient situations, which can normalize behavior for short periods of time. The evaluation of current symptoms should therefore be based on accounts of behavior and reports of ADHD symptoms during a typical day in the life of the patient.

Obtaining accurate accounts of attention deficit hyperactivity disorder symptoms

One difficulty of diagnosing ADHD is that adult informants tend to minimize their symptoms. Adults may also have only a poor recall of their symptoms and behaviors as children. It is also not unusual to find a patient who appears too eager to be diagnosed with ADHD and perceives the diagnosis as a solution to problems that are unrelated to ADHD. The diagnosis of ADHD can nevertheless be established in most cases by:

- accurate use of the DSM-IV criteria;
- enquiring after detailed accounts of problems related to ADHD symptoms;
- obtaining collateral information from relatives, partners, or work colleagues whenever possible;
- review of written reports (eg, school or work reports) whenever possible.

Compensatory mechanisms reduce apparent impairments

Adults have a degree of control over their circumstances and often modify their life to compensate for or minimize impairments related to ADHD. Hyperactivity may be managed by choosing an occupation that keeps people on their feet and moving around; impulsivity may be better adapted to a job that requires prompt action without excessive planning; and inattentiveness may be dealt with by adopting a freelance occupation in which people can control their own schedule. The fact that some people are successful in one of life's realms, such as the workplace and career, does not preclude the possibility of a diagnosis, since they may be impaired in other ways.

The clinician therefore needs to understand and enquire about what compensating strategies may be in use. Although such strategies may be highly successful in a few cases, they often come at a personal cost in terms of distress from the symptoms and the constant effort that is needed to compensate adequately. Common compensatory mechanisms include:

- support by a member of the family or paid assistant;
- support of an organized partner;
- flexible work schedule;
- occupations or activities where impulsivity may be a positive factor or where high levels of risk may be involved (eg, emergency services, adventure sports);
- excessive preplanning and checking to compensate for difficulties in organizing, planning ahead, and forgetfulness;
- use of electronic aids such as smart phones with alarms, reminders, and electronic calendars.

ADHD has a very wide range of presentations and impairments from mild to very severe. In the most severe cases, adults with ADHD are unable to function in work and have very poorly developed social lives. They may present with extreme levels of impulsivity, emotional dysregulation, distractibility, and poor organization that severely impairs their ability to cope with activities of everyday life. On the other hand, some individuals with ADHD are high functioning and can manage most aspects of their daily lives, but present with a range of mild but persistent symptoms and impairments. Some typical presenting complaints in people meeting clinical criteria for ADHD that responded to treatment are listed in Table 4.2.

Diagnostic protocol

The UK Adult ADHD Network (UKAAN) recommends a standard diagnostic protocol that can be widely adopted in clinical practice. Use of this diagnostic protocol will establish basic procedures, provide a minimum standard, and enable comparative studies across sites that adopt the protocol. Using a standard protocol will help in the development of the

Examples of presenting complaints of adults who met DSM-IV criteria for attention deficit hyperactivity disorder and showed good response to treatment

26-year-old female: Disorganized. Unable to work. Had ceaseless mental activity and difficulty shopping. Treated for anxiety and depression. Used cannabis to "calm thoughts." Cares for two children that have ADHD

22-year-old male: Unable to cope at college. Has had to repeat his first year of college for third year in a row, despite a high IQ, high motivation, a supportive family, and good level of education

18-year-old male: IQ of approximately 70. Had behavioral problems at home. Lacked insight. Engaged in binge drinking. Main presenting complaint was extreme irritability and aggression

30-year-old female: Experienced irritable and volatile moods. Treated for depression. Managed to get through college but had to expend significantly more energy and put in far more effort than equivalents in her peer group, due to difficulties coping with inattention, distractibility, and planning

25-year-old male: Unemployed and stayed at home doing very little. Complained of severe inner restlessness. Was unable to focus on a task for more than a few minutes. Grossly distractible and had unfocused thought processes

35-year-old male: Displayed extreme impulsivity. Physically and verbally aggressive. Engaged in binge drinking of alcohol on a regular basis and often got into fights in public drinking establishments

Table 4.2 Examples of presenting complaints of adults who met DSM-IV criteria for attention deficit hyperactivity disorder and showed good response to treatment.
ADHD, attention deficit hyperactivity disorder; DSM-IV, Diagnostic and Statistical Manual of Mental Disorders, fourth edition; IQ, intelligence quotient.

clinical skills required to diagnose ADHD in adults, by linking the protocol to training programs and sharing of expertise between clinicians.

Development of a standard protocol is not intended to change clinical practice for specialists who have already established their own valid diagnostic methods. However, the recommended protocol uses screening and diagnostic instruments that have been widely adopted in Europe and are used by many experienced clinicians. The diagnostic instruments for this protocol were selected on the basis of their widespread use, previous validation, and being freely available. All materials are provided in the Appendix can also be downloaded from www.ukaan.org.

It is envisaged that ongoing developments in the field will lead to modifications of this protocol, as diagnostic criteria and improved instruments are developed. UKAAN have kept the protocol to the minimum required to evaluate the diagnosis and its treatment outcomes. As such, this section is not a comprehensive review of all available assessments tools.

The minimum protocol for the clinical evaluation of ADHD in adults includes the following components:

- a physician's referral form (Appendix I);
- screening questionnaires (Appendix A; Appendices C–F);
- scales for assessment of current symptoms (Appendix A; Appendix C; Appendix F);
- scales for assessment of retrospective (childhood) symptoms (Appendix D; Appendix E);
- evaluation of impairment (Appendix J);
- evaluation of comorbidity (Appendix K);
- diagnostic interview (Appendix G).

Physician's referral form

Physician referral forms should include all relevant medical information with special attention to the following:

- history of brain trauma or injury;
- history of cardiovascular disease, with particular attention to dysrhythmia and a family history of sudden death. If the patient has a positive history of cardiovascular disease or any cardiac abnormalities detected on physical examination, a recent ECG should be included (Appendix H);
- recent physical examination;
- history of drug use and dependency;
- history of medical disorders;
- history of psychiatric and behavioral problems with particular attention to comorbid conditions such as:
  - anxiety or depression
  - bipolar affective disorder
  - schizophrenia or other psychotic disorders
  - obsessive-compulsive disorder
  - personality disorder
  - pervasive developmental disorder (eg, autism spectrum disorder)
  - substance abuse or addiction disorders
  - antisocial behavior and forensic history.

Screening questionnaires

There are several screening tools that have been developed for ADHD. UKAAN recommends the use of symptoms checklists for the 18 DSM-IV items; for example, the Adult ADHD Self Report Scale (ASRS) and Barkley's adult ADHD symptoms checklist.

Adult ADHD Self Report Scale

The Adult ADHD Self Report Scale (ASRS) screening tool (Appendix A), validated by the World Health Organization (WHO) [3], is one of the most widely used in recent epidemiological studies. It covers each of the 18 items for the DSM-IV, but has reworded each item to better reflect the way that the symptoms affect adults. In addition to this, a short, six-item version has high sensitivity to the clinical diagnosis and can be used as a brief screening tool in primary care, or in a busy clinical setting.

Barkley's adult ADHD symptoms checklist

The Barkley's adult ADHD symptoms checklist is a simple screening tool that systematically enquires after each of the DSM-IV symptoms for ADHD [4]. The scale can be used for evaluation of clinical outcome following treatment.

Diagnostic interviews
The Diagnostic Interview for ADHD in Adults

The Diagnostic Interview for ADHD in Adults (DIVA) is a diagnostic interview for the diagnosis of ADHD in adults, developed by Kooij and Francken from the Netherlands [5] (Appendix G). A PDF of the DIVA interview and all instructions for use of the diagnostic interview can be downloaded from www.divacenter.eu and an iphone/ipad/android app will be available. The DIVA interview was developed because there was a need for a structured diagnostic interview for ADHD in adults that is easily available at low cost and has been translated into several languages for both clinical and research assessments. The DIVA interview investigates the DSM criteria for ADHD in childhood using retrospective accounts and current symptoms in adults, and links this information to impairments in five areas of function:

- work/education;
- relationships/family;
- social contacts;
- free time/hobbies;
- self-confidence/self-image.

Examples are provided for ADHD in adults and children that are sensitive to the developmental stage and provide a guide for probe questions to patients during the interview, if required. The interview starts with assessment of inattention, continues with hyperactivity-impulsivity, and finishes with the assessment of impairment. The DIVA interview takes approximately 60 minutes to complete in most cases.

Connors Adult ADHD Diagnostic Interview for DSM-IV

The Connors Adult ADHD Diagnostic Interview for DSM-IV (CAADID) [6] is a semi-structured interview that has been frequently used to confirm the diagnosis of ADHD in adults for pharmacological studies. It has two main parts: the first part collects background information about the clinical and developmental history and is not essential to the formal diagnosis, but is a very useful guide for clinicians new to the diagnosis of ADHD; the second part systematically addresses each of the 18 DSM-IV items for current and retrospective (childhood) symptoms and impairments due to ADHD. CAADID is not free to use, which limits its routine use in clinical practice.

Attention deficit hyperactivity disorder rating scales

There are several rating scales available for the evaluation of ADHD in adults. While some focus on the DSM-IV items, others include additional symptoms and impairments that are commonly found in adults with ADHD. For the minimum protocol, UKAAN recommends focusing on the 18 DSM-IV items for current and retrospective symptoms (eg, using the ASRS or the Barkley scale).

Assessment of ADHD should include at least one rating scale for adult symptoms and one for retrospective (childhood) symptoms. In both cases, information should be obtained from the patient and from an external informant (usually a parent or older relative for childhood ratings; a parent, partner, or close friend for current ratings) whenever possible (Table 4.3) (Appendix C–F).

Evaluation of impairment
Weiss Functional Impairment Rating Scale
Impairment is a key part of the diagnostic algorithm and an important outcome measure. UKAAN therefore recommend the use of a detailed rating scale that captures the types of impairment that are commonly seen in adults with ADHD. The Weiss Functional Impairment Rating Scale was developed for this purpose and is now widely used [7] (Appendix B). The scale consists of 72 items covering the following domains of impairment:
- family;
- work;
- school/college;
- life skills;
- social functioning;
- self-concept;
- risk taking.

Barkley Functional Impairment Scale
Because in practice it may not always be possible to include such a long scale for the evaluation of impairment within a standard clinic protocol, an alternative to the Weiss scale is to use the ten summary items from

Recommended rating scale measures of attention deficit hyperactivity disorder symptoms
Self-ratings of current ADHD symptoms: ASRS or Barkley scale
Informant ratings of current ADHD symptoms: Barkley scale
Self-ratings of childhood ADHD symptoms: Barkley scale
Informant ratings of childhood ADHD symptoms: Barkley scale

Table 4.3 Recommended rating scale measures of attention deficit hyperactivity disorder symptoms. ADHD, attention deficit hyperactivity disorder; ASRS, Adult ADHD Self Rating Scale.

the Barkley scale [4]. These address whether the patient has impairment related to the symptoms of ADHD in the following areas:

- in the home with the immediate family;
- in work or occupation;
- social interaction with others;
- activities or dealings with the community;
- any educational activities;
- dating or marital relationship;
- money management;
- driving a motor vehicle;
- leisure or recreational activities;
- management of daily responsibilities.

Comorbidity

Evaluating comorbidity is a time-consuming but essential part of any diagnostic assessment for ADHD. In clinical practice, it is not usually possible to include a standardized diagnostic instrument for adult mental health disorders in addition to the systematic evaluation of ADHD symptoms. Furthermore, the available diagnostic instruments are not designed to differentiate symptoms of ADHD that overlap with diagnostic criteria for other common mental health disorders, such as depressive episodes and bipolar disorder. UKAAN therefore only recommends the use of a standardized clinical interview for adult psychiatric disorders when this is needed for research.

For the minimum protocol, it is essential that common adult mental health disorders that either co-occur at increased rates in ADHD or may be part of the differential diagnosis are carefully evaluated. The assessment of comorbidity is usually completed by a trained psychiatrist or a specialist in the diagnosis of adult mental health disorders. UKAAN recommends the use of a standard diagnostic checklist for the inclusion and exclusion of the following key disorders (Appendix K):

- bipolar affective disorder;
- major depression;
- anxiety disorder;
- obsessive–compulsive disorder;

- schizophrenia;
- substance abuse disorder;
- addiction;
- borderline personality disorder;
- antisocial personality disorder;
- other personality disorder;
- tic disorder;
- autism spectrum disorder;
- learning disability (general);
- specific reading difficulty (dyslexia);
- specific mathematics difficulty.

References

1   Asherson P. Clinical assessment and treatment of attention deficit hyperactivity disorder in adults. *Expert Rev Neurother.* 2005;5:525-539.
2   World Health Organization. *The ICD-10 Classification of Mental and Behavioural Disorders.* Geneva: World Health Organization;2002. Accessed August 25, 2012.
3   Kessler RC, Adler L, Ames M, et al. The World Health Organization Adult ADHD Self-Report Scale (ASRS). *Psychol Med.* 2005;35:245-256.
4   Barkley MA, Murphy RA. Attention-Deficit Hyperactivity Disorder: a Clinical Workbook. Third ed. New York: Guildford Press; 2006.
5   Kooij JJS, Francken MH. Diagnostic Interview for ADHD Adults (DIVA scale). DIVA Foundation website. www.ukaan.org/clinicians_resource.htm. Accessed August 25, 2012.
6   Epstein JN, Kollins SH. Psychometric properties of an adult ADHD diagnostic interview. *J Atten Disord.* 2006;9:504-514.
7   Weiss Scale. www.caddra.ca/cms4/pdfs/caddraGuidelines2011WFIRS_S.pdf. Accessed August 25, 2012.

Chapter 5

Neuropsychological assessment

The potential contribution of neuropsychological assessment to the diagnostic assessment of attention deficit hyperactivity disorder (ADHD) of
is limited by a number of factors, including:

- Specific cognitive deficits identified by neuropsychological
  testing have not been established as a specific marker of ADHD [1].
  While the absence of cognitive deficits will not reject the diagnosis,
  the presence of cognitive deficits can be explained by different
  underlying problems or pathology (eg, anxiety, learning disability).
- ADHD diagnosis is made based upon behavioral evidence.
  However, cognitive deficits do not necessarily transfer to behavior,
  as an individual may have acquired good adaptive functioning
  through the development of compensatory strategies.
- The high risk of false-negatives limits the validity of tests in clinical
  practice. People with ADHD may do well on novel tasks and/or
  on tasks conducted in an optimal environment (ie, a medical clinic
  or study center), which helps them to concentrate better. In this
  setting, they generally will receive structure, encouragement,
  and feedback from the tester, which is a motivating factor.
- The heterogeneity of ADHD criteria and inconsistent assessment
  methodologies used across research studies makes it difficult to
  draw firm conclusions.

UKAAN, *Handbook for Attention Deficit Hyperactivity
Disorder in Adults*, DOI: 10.1007/978-1-908517-79-1_5,
© Springer Healthcare 2013

Notwithstanding these caveats, a neuropsychological assessment can be useful to support a clinical diagnosis of ADHD by providing helpful additional information. Task performance can be compared with normative data to provide information about the severity of performance deficits in an easy to understand form (eg, by determining percentile ranks). In this way, valuable clinical information can be obtained about an individual's cognitive strengths and weaknesses.

This may be particularly helpful in certain circumstances and settings, as it provides a functional expectation or hypotheses regarding the individual's ability to perform in daily activities (eg, academic, occupational, and/or domestic tasks) and from which discrepancies may be identified in performance across different aspects of functioning. For the same reasons, a neuropsychological assessment can greatly assist, for example, in the overall assessment of defendants with ADHD when preparing reports for court proceedings [2]. It can also be helpful to establish IQ to identify patients in whom this is lower than required for their work level and who presume the reason for their work failure is due to ADHD; or where patients with a higher IQ than required are not coping at work because of impairments directly related to ADHD.

Neuropsychological testing is specifically indicated in cases where there is evidence of significant learning disability or unexplained 'patchy' cognitive abilities. It is also helpful where there is a history suggestive of specific brain injury or damage (eg, secondary to traumatic head injury or encephalitis). Testing should also be considered where the impairment at work, school, or home is greater than would normally be expected by ADHD symptoms alone.

Neuropsychological tests

Meta-analyses have indicated that a broad range of neuropsychological tests show significant deficits in adults with ADHD [1,3]. Key tests to assess cognitive function in adults with ADHD include tests of intelligence, attention, and impulsivity (Table 5.1 and Table 5.2). It is important to observe an individual's behavior during testing and note any behavioral manifestations of symptoms, such as inattention (eg, need for repetition of instructions, distraction by external stimuli, omission of items on

Neuropsychological tests used to assess cognitive function in attention deficit hyperactivity disorder adults in a clinical setting

Cognitive function	Test
Intelligence quotient (IQ)	Wechsler Adult Intelligence Scale: • Digit-symbol coding • Arithmetic • Block design • Digit span
Attention	Letter cancellation test
	Trail making test
	Test of Everyday Attention: • Map search • Telephone search whilst counting • Visual elevator • Lottery
	Continuous performance test omission errors
Impulsivity and disinhibition	Matching familiar figures test
	Stroop Neuropsychological Screening test
	Continuous performance test commission errors

Table 5.1 Neuropsychological tests used to assess cognitive function in attention deficit hyperactivity disorder adults in a clinical setting.

Neuropsychological tests commonly used in the assessment of attention deficit hyperactivity disorder adults in a clinical setting

Test	Description of test
Letter Cancellation Test*	Test of selective attention. Testee has to strike out one letter from a range of alphabetical letters with both speed and accuracy. The number of lines completed and number/percentage of errors is recorded
Trail Making Test	Test of scanning and visuo-motor tracking, divided attention, and cognitive flexibility. Test is given in two parts: A and B. Part A involves connecting consecutively numbered circles on one work sheet, and then connecting consecutively numbered and lettered circles by alternating between the two sequences (eg, 1 to A to 2 to B to 3 to C and so on). Errors are usually pointed out as they occur and the time to complete each part is scored (age-adjusted norms are available). Disproportionately poor performance on Part B (eg, 3x slower on Part B than Part A) indicates problems with self-monitoring
Map Search (TEA)	Test of selective attention. Testee has to search for symbols (eg, for a knife and fork sign representing eating facilities) on a color map of the Philadelphia area. The score is the number out of 80 found in 2 minutes

Table 5.2 Neuropsychological tests commonly used in the assessment of attention deficit hyperactivity disorder adults in a clinical setting (continues overleaf).

Test	Description of test
Telephone Search Whilst Counting (TEA)	Test of divided and sustained attention. Testee has to listen and count strings of tones in a series played on a disk while simultaneously working on another task that requires them to look for key symbols whilst searching through a telephone directory. A 'dual task decrement' is calculated by following a scoring procedure set out in the manual
Visual Elevator (TEA)	Test of attentional switching and cognitive flexibility. Testee has to count up and down as she/he follows a series of visually presented 'floors' in an elevator. Direction of counting is indicated by arrows, which are reversed at intermittent intervals. Accuracy and timing scores are calculated
Lottery (TEA)	Test of sustained attention that requires the testee to listen out for winning lottery numbers from a presentation of a 10-minute series of audio-presented numbers. An accuracy score is calculated
Continuous Performance Test (omission errors and commission errors)*	Test of vigilance (ie, ability to sustain and focus attention, and inhibit a response). Usually a monotonous task presented on a computer. The test typically involves the sequential presentation of stimuli (eg, strings of letters or numbers) over a period of time with instructions to indicate (eg, press key on keyboard) when a target stimulus is perceived. Target stimuli are presented with a low target frequency. Duration of task varies but is usually at least 8 minutes. Mean reaction time and error scores are recorded. Missed targets (false negatives) represent errors of omission and are associated with ability to sustain attention. Mistaken targets (false positives) are errors of commission and associated with ability to inhibit a response
Matching Familiar Figures Test	Test of response inhibition. Testee has to identify target pictures among five distractors with both speed and accuracy. Scores are recorded for mean reaction time and number of errors
Stroop Neuropsychological Screening Test	Test of response inhibition. Test is presented in two trials, one requiring the testee to read color words printed in ink of different colors (ie, generating a pre-potent response). The second part requires the testee to name the printed colors. The stroop effect is a markedly slowed naming response due to distraction from the color-word interference trial when a color name is printed in ink of a different colour. Time and errors are scored

Table 5.2 Neuropsychological tests commonly used in the assessment of attention deficit hyperactivity disorder adults in a clinical setting (continued). TEA, Test of Everyday Attention. *For norms, see [12,13]; for all other norms refer to test manuals.

questionnaires, daydreaming); hyperactivity (eg, fidgeting, restlessness, foot tapping, leg shaking, fiddling with papers); or impulsivity (eg, prematurely responding on timed tests, blurting out irrelevant questions or answers, rapid shifts in topic of conversation).

Intelligence

Although people with ADHD often underachieve, it is important to determine their intellectual function, as this will provide an indication of their potential and ensure that achievement levels are put into perspective. A crude indicator of this would be to compare their occupational and academic attainment with that of sibling achievement.

Intellectual measures that have been shown to highlight ADHD in adults are tasks that rely heavily on working memory and processing speed abilities (eg, subtests of the Wechsler Adult Intelligence Scale [WAIS], digit-symbol coding, arithmetic, block design, and digit span) [3,4]. However, ADHD symptoms may result in artificially low IQ scores due to inattentive and/or impulsive responding [5]. Memory deficits have been reported in adults with ADHD [6] and may play an important role in some of the most common impairments seen in adults with ADHD, such as forgetfulness, disorganization, and planning. A benefit of using the WAIS is that in addition to giving an overall assessment of intelligence, it can also give an index of working memory functioning.

Attention

Attentional functions are usually subdivided into different domains, including selective attention, divided attention, shifting attention, and sustained attention. A useful clinical test battery is the Test of Everyday Attention [TEA], which was devised to include ecologically valid 'real life' tasks [7].

Selective attention is the ability to focus attention on one stimulus source and screen out distracting irrelevant stimuli. This can be assessed using the Letter Cancellation Test [8] and the Map Search subtest of the TEA battery [7].

Divided attention is the ability to attend to two or more stimuli simultaneously. This can be assessed using the Telephone Search Whilst Counting sub test of the TEA battery [7].

Shifting attention is the ability to switch attention between two or more sources of information. This can be assessed using Part B of the Trail Making Test [9,10], and the Visual Elevator subtest from the TEA battery [7].

Sustained attention is the ability to maintain attention over a long period of time with only a limited frequency of reinforcement. This can be assessed by omission errors recorded by Continuous Performance Tests [8]. The Lottery subtest of the TEA battery is also a sustained attention task [7].

Impulsivity and disinhibition

Response inhibition is an executive function or 'higher order' cognitive process. Impaired response inhibition reduces an individual's ability to control either actions or speech. It means that an individual has difficulty applying the 'brakes' to halt an inappropriate response. Tests that are helpful to assess disinhibition include commission errors recorded by Continuous Performance Tests [8], the Matching Familiar Figures test [11–13], and the Stroop test [14,15]. This may also be expressed as a planning deficit [16].

Case studies

Case study #1 of a patient with suspected attention deficit hyperactivity disorder

Mr Jones was 32 years old when referred for an ADHD assessment. He had been experiencing great difficulties at work, where he was employed as a clerical assistant in an office. He said that he had always had difficulty with organization and completing administrative tasks, but that it had become worse in the past few years. More recently, he had been avoiding communicating by email as he found it particularly stressful and time-consuming to correspond this way. These problems were discussed with him in his annual appraisal, resulting in him being referred for an occupational health assessment. During the assessment, he became distressed and tearful when talking about his current work situation. Mr Jones was not taking any prescribed medication at the time of the assessment and described himself as a 'social drinker' without a history of substance use. Aside from an interview about his functioning in childhood and adulthood, the following test results were obtained:

- **WAIS-III IQ:** full-scale IQ score=105; performance IQ score=102; verbal IQ score=106;
- **Barkley ADHD Behavior Scale:** childhood symptom score=27 (standardized score=0.93), (6 inattentive – 1 impulsive-hyperactive); current ADHD symptoms score=35 (standardized score=2.95), (9 inattentive – 4 impulsive-hyperactive);

- **Letter Cancellation Test:** 14 lines completed (standardized score= 0.58); 0% errors (standardized score=0.75);
- **Continuous Performance Test:** mean reaction time=1.10 seconds (standardized score=2.87); errors of omission=0 (standardized score=0.46); errors of commission=0 (standardized score=0.40);
- **Matching Familiar Figure Test:** mean reaction time=32 seconds (standardized score=2.73); errors=3 (standardized score=0.42);
- **Hospital Anxiety and Depression Scale (HADS):** anxiety=14; depression=13.

The retrospective ratings on the Barkley Behavior Scale did not strongly indicate a DSM-IV diagnosis of ADHD in childhood (ie, a standard deviation of 0.93). Mr Jones's general intellectual abilities fell within the normal range. This was generally consistent with his description of his childhood (eg, the absence of behavioral problems). He described himself as an anxious child. He left school at 16 years of age after obtaining six low-to-mid range General Certificates of Secondary Education (GCSEs).

In adulthood, Mr Jones rated his symptoms on the Barkley Current Behavior Scale to have considerably worsened and rated these symptoms to cause him impairment in many domains. His performance on neuropsychological testing, however, indicated his tendency to favor accuracy over speed. His performance was slow, careful, and considered, and he made no errors.

Mr Jones obtained high ratings of anxiety and depression on the HADS, and this was supported by an assessment of his current mental state.

Overall, Mr Jones appeared to have had an anxious predisposition from childhood. His attention problems were most likely a feature of underlying anxiety and mood disorders, rather than ADHD. In the interview, Mr Jones described himself to have some obsessive and perfectionist characteristics and it is likely that he set himself high standards at work that were unrealistic to achieve. He presented with low self esteem and lacking in confidence, and this seemed to relate to him experiencing a sequence of negative life events over the past few years (eg, car accident, divorce, occupational problems). Mr Jones was referred for cognitive behavioral therapy for anxiety management and directed to some reading material on the topic.

Case study #2 of a patient with suspected attention deficit hyperactivity disorder

Mr Blake was 20 years old when referred for an ADHD assessment. He had scraped through his first year at university after having to re-sit two examinations. He had 10 GCSEs and three A levels at grade B. He had failed his first second-year university assessment and he had been told by tutors that he was disorganized and his written work was unacceptable. He had a fiery temperament and had fallen out with his personal tutor and fellow students. In an interview with his mother, it was learned that at age 11 years he had been assessed by an educational psychologist and was diagnosed with ADHD and dyslexia. His mother had refused treatment with medication and they had disengaged from services. In the past, his parents had supported him greatly in his studies by providing structure, time-tabling deadlines, and checking his work. He was now living away from home. Mr Blake presented as a somewhat intense and excitable young man, who would lose his train of thought and flit from one subject to another. During neuropsychological testing, he did not easily follow test instructions and these had to be repeated to ensure he understood the task. It was noted that he became quickly distracted by people talking outside the window. Mr Blake was not taking any prescribed medication at the time of the assessment and he admitted to drinking around 20 units of beer a week and using cannabis two or three times per week, which he said helped him relax in the evenings. Aside from an interview about his functioning in childhood and adulthood, the following test results were obtained:

- **WAIS-III IQ:** full-scale IQ score=113; performance IQ score=108; verbal IQ score=114;
- **Barkley ADHD Behavior Scale:** childhood symptom score=39 (standardized score=1.52), (6 inattentive – 7 impulsive-hyperactive); current ADHD symptoms score=29 (standardized score=1.64), (6 inattentive – 4 impulsive-hyperactive);
- **Letter Cancellation Test:** 21 lines completed (standardized score=2.95); errors=41% (standardized score=6.34);

- **Continuous Performance Test:** mean reaction time=0.68 seconds (standardized score=0.06); errors of omission=6 (standardized score=3.51); errors of commission=8 (standardized score=3.25);
- **Matching Familiar Figure Test:** mean reaction time=7 seconds (standardized score=–1.37); errors=13 (standardized score=2.74);
- **HADS:** anxiety=11; depression=9.

Mr Blake had a full-scale IQ score of 113 which fell in the high average range of general intellectual ability. There was considerable subtest scatter and subtests that load on working memory (and require concentration) were significantly lower than Mr Blake's average verbal score. His academic attainment at university was considerably lower than expected from his intellectual ability.

The retrospective ratings on the Barkley Behavior Scales were consistent with childhood ADHD, as was his mother's account of his behavior in childhood, and him receiving an ADHD diagnosis at age 11 years. This was also supported by secondary school reports provided by his mother. In adulthood, Mr Blake rated himself to continue having ADHD symptoms (both attention and hyperactivity-impulsivity) on the Barkley Current Behavior Scale and in the interview he explained how these impact on his daily activities at a level of impairment. His self-reported account was consistent with his performance on neuropsychological testing, which indicated significant problems with attentional control and impulsivity.

Mr Blake obtained ratings on the HADS that indicated the presence of anxiety and mild depressive symptoms. However, this was not supported by a brief mental state examination and these ratings may have reflected lability of mood and a difficulty with self-regulation. Nevertheless, Mr Blake reported long-standing feelings of frustration over not achieving his personal potential and concerns about his ability to complete his second year at university; thus, anxiety may have been a secondary comorbid condition. Mr Blake was prescribed medication and given psychoeducational materials. Following liaison with the university, it was recommended that lengthy examinations be partitioned into smaller 'chunks' that he could sit independently. In addition, Mr Blake was allowed 25% additional time for examinations and 10 minutes rest time per hour.

References

1   Bálint S, Czobor P, Komlósi S, Mészáros Á, Simon S, Bitter I. Attention deficit hyperactivity disorder (ADHD): gender- and age-related differences in neurocognition. *Psychol Med.* 2009;39:1337-1345.

2   Young S. Attention Deficit Hyperactivity Disorder. In: Young S, Kopelman M, Gudjonsson G, eds, *Forensic Neuropsychology In Practice: A Guide to Assessment and Legal Processes.* New York, NY: Oxford University Press; 2009:81-107.

3   Hervey AS, Epstein JN, Curry JF. Neuropsychology of adults with attention-deficit/ hyperactivity disorder: a meta-analytic review. *Neuropsychology.* 2004, 18:485-503.

4   Quinlan DM. Assesment of attention deficit/hyperactivity disorder and comorbities. In: TE Brown, ed, *Attention-Deficit Disorders and Comorbidity in Children, Adolescents, and Adults.* Washington DC: American Psychiatric Press; 2001.

5   Gudjonsson G, Young S. An overlooked vulnerability in a defendant: attention deficit hyperactivity disorder (ADHD) and a miscarriage of justice. *Legal and Criminological Psychology.* 2006;11:211-218.

6   Young S, Morris RG, Toone BK, Tyson C. Spatial working memory and strategy formation in adults diagnosed with attention deficit hyperactivity disorder. *Pers Individ Dif.* 2006;41:653-661.

7   Roberston IH, Ward T, Ridgeway V, Nimmo-Smith I. *The Test of Everyday Attention.* Bury St Edmunds: Thames Valley Test; 1994.

8   Lezak MD, Howieson DB, Loring DW. *Neuropsychological Assessment.* 4th ed. Oxford: Oxford University Press; 2004.

9   Reitan RM. Validity of the trail making test as an indicator of organic brain damage. *Percept Mot Skills.* 1958;8:271-276.

10 Spreen O, Strauss E. *A Compendium of Neuropsychological Tests.* New York, NY: Oxford University Press; 1998.

11 Cairnes E, Cammock T. Development of a more reliable version of the Matching Familiar Figures Test. *Dev Psychol.* 1978:14:555-556.

12 Young S, Channon S, Toone BK. Neuropsychological assessment of attention deficit hyperactivity disorder in adulthood. *Clin Neuropsychol Assess.* 2000;1:283-294.

13 Young S, Gudjonsson G. Neurospychological correlates of the YAQ-S self-reported ADHD symptomatology, emotional and social problems, and delinquent behaviours. *Br J Psychiatry.* 2005;44:47-57.

14 Trenerry MR, Crosson B, DeBoe J, Leber WR. *Stroop Neuropsychological Screening Test Manual.* Odessa, FL: Psychological Assessment Resources; 1989.

15 Young S, Morris RG, Bramham J, Tyson C. Inhibitory dysfunction on the Stroop in adults diagnosed with attention deficit hyperactivity disorder. *Pers Individ Dif.* 2006;41:1377-1384.

16 Young S, Morris RG, Toone BK, Tyson, C. Planning ability in adults diagnosed with attention-deficit/hyperactivity disorder: A deficit in planning ability. *Neuropsychology.* 2007;21: 581-589.

Chapter 6

Comorbid symptoms, syndromes, and disorders

Clinical implications

Co-occurring symptoms, syndromes, and disorders are the rule rather than the exception in adults (and children) with attention deficit hyperactivity disorder (ADHD). A careful clinical evaluation is therefore needed that includes a full developmental and psychiatric history and mental state examination. The key features that discriminate ADHD symptoms from those of other disorders include:

- specific clusters of inattentive, hyperactive, and impulsive symptoms;
- childhood or early adolescent onset with chronic trait-like course;
- lack of a clear distinction from the premorbid mental state;
- nonepisodic nature of the symptoms.

The core operational symptoms that formally define ADHD should be systematically evaluated and their lifetime course and relationship to other symptoms explored. In principle, ADHD is no more difficult to diagnose than other common mental health problems such as anxiety and depression, but clinicians must be aware of the typical onset, course and nature of ADHD symptoms. Further guidance on distinguishing ADHD from specific disorders and treating ADHD when it co-occurs with other mental health disorders is provided in this chapter.

UKAAN, *Handbook for Attention Deficit Hyperactivity Disorder in Adults*, DOI: 10.1007/978-1-908517-79-1_6, © Springer Healthcare 2013

Sources of comorbid symptoms, syndromes, and disorders

Comorbidities in ADHD fall into three main categories that each have different implications for treatment:

- symptoms that form part of the core ADHD syndrome but are not listed within current operational criteria;
- overlapping neurodevelopmental disorders and traits that share etiological influences with ADHD;
- disorders that develop from the psychosocial consequences of ADHD or are driven by core features of the disorder such as impulsivity.

Core symptoms not listed within current operational criteria

Behaviors that reflect executive functions

Several authors describe a broad range of symptoms and behaviors that are commonly found in adults who fulfill the diagnostic criteria for ADHD and are thought to represent core features of the condition. Of these, behavioral symptoms that are thought to reflect impairments in executive functions have been highlighted as central to ADHD and may be particularly sensitive and specific to the underlying disorder [1–3]. While these may not always be seen in direct tests of cognitive function (eg, response inhibition, planning tasks) and etiological models continue to be hotly debated, performance deficits are usually seen in the way that people with ADHD manage daily tasks [1,2]. Problems reported by adults with ADHD that may reflect executive dysfunction deficits include: impaired self-organization, attentional and emotional regulation, sustained effort, and alertness (see Chapter 2).

Emotional lability

Emotional lability is a common co-occurring feature of ADHD, described in DSM-IV as an associated feature of the disorder. The characteristics in adults with ADHD consists of irritable or angry moods, with volatile and changeable emotions, where emotional changes are short-lived and generally reactive to the environment, shifting from normal mood to depression or mild excitement [4]. Although it has been noted since the earliest conceptualizations of ADHD [5,6], emotional lability is considered an associated feature of the condition, rather than a core component of the condition itself.

There is an ongoing controversy about the relationship between emotional lability and ADHD in children and young adolescents, particularly the question of whether symptoms of bipolar spectrum disorder, when they co-occur with ADHD, represent symptoms of ADHD itself or are a separate co-occurring disorder requiring additional treatment [7]. There is also overlap with the type of emotional instability seen in borderline personality disorder.

However, most clinical experts working with adults with ADHD are in agreement that emotional lability is a common symptom that frequently responds to drug treatments for ADHD, including stimulants and atomoxetine [8,9]. In a trial of methylphenidate by Reimherr and colleagues [9], it was observed that during the course of the treatment response, symptoms reflecting emotional dysregulation correlated with response of attention and distractibility (R=0.88) and hyperactivity-impulsivity (R=0.81). These findings, and more recent studies by Rosler and colleagues [10], show that in adults with ADHD there are similar effects sizes for stimulants on symptoms of emotional lability, as those for the core syndrome of ADHD.

Symptoms of attention deficit hyperactivity disorder that mimic other disorders

There are a range of symptoms and behaviors of ADHD that can be mistaken for symptoms of other common mental health disorders such as anxiety, depression, and personality disorder. It is therefore important when evaluating the potential role of comorbidities that a careful account is taken of the mental state and precise description of the mental phenomena and their onset and course. Examples of symptoms that may mimic other disorders include the following:

- mind wandering and ceaseless unfocused mental activity may be mistaken for anxious worrying;
- avoidance of certain situations may be mistaken for phobic responses:
  - avoidance of shops because of dislike of waiting in queues
  - avoidance of travel due to forgetfulness and difficulty in planning

- avoidance of social situations because of difficulty in focusing on conversations, or problems resulting from an impulsive style of social interaction
- impulsivity, mood instability, and difficulties with relationships may be mistaken for a personality disorder;
- low self esteem, mood instability, and initial insomnia may be mistaken for depression;
- restlessness, irritability, over-talking, and ceaseless, unfocused thought processes may be mistaken for hypomania.

Neurodevelopmental disorders and overlapping etiological influences

It has long been recognized that symptoms of ADHD often occur alongside other neurodevelopmental disorders and traits, including general cognitive ability (low IQ), autism spectrum disorders (ASD), specific reading difficulties (dyslexia), and motor coordination disorders (dyspraxia).

The association between ADHD and a lower IQ has not been fully evaluated in adults. In children, there is only a weak association of ADHD with low IQ [11]. ADHD should not be viewed as a learning disability, as the distribution of IQ in people with ADHD spans the entire range and is only slightly different from that seen in the general population. This means that for the large majority of cases, ADHD in adults should be managed by general adult mental health services in collaboration with primary care, rather than special needs or learning disability services.

The overlap of ADHD with autism is interesting because, according to current diagnostic criteria, ADHD should not be diagnosed in the presence of ASD [12,13]. However, it is now clear that ADHD and ASD frequently co-occur. As a result, clinical guidelines are explicit in clarifying that ADHD should be diagnosed and treated in the presence of ASD, and that ASD should not trump the diagnosis of ADHD but rather should be treated as a common co-occuring disorder [12].

The reason for the frequent co-occurrence of ADHD with other neurodevelopmental disorders and traits is thought to be a result of shared etiological influences, particularly genetic risk factors. There are a number of twin studies that demonstrate the overlap of genetic influences between

ADHD and ASD, as well as dyslexia and motor coordination difficulties [14,15]. These studies suggest that the genes involved have pleiotropic effects. This means that genetic variation within individual genes or sets of genes have multiple developmental outcomes.

Recognition of co-occurring neurodevelopmental disorders is important because these would not be expected to respond directly to drug treatments for ADHD and may be a source of continued impairment, even if there is a good response of ADHD symptoms to drug treatments. Clinical evaluation of ADHD should therefore include a screen for other neurodevelopmental problems that may form an important part of the clinical picture and may be a source of continued, potentially lifelong, impairments.

Attention deficit hyperactivity disorder as a risk factor for other mental health disorders and behavioral problems

ADHD is associated with the development of additional behavioral and psychiatric problems including antisocial behavior, substance use disorders, anxiety, depression, and personality disorder. The causal links between ADHD and these disorders and behavioral problems are complex and include both genetic and environmental influences.

Conduct problems

Longitudinal studies find that ADHD may be a precursor for the development of conduct problems and this in turn may lead to conduct disorder and persistence of antisocial behavior in to adult life. Quantitative genetic analyses suggest that the overlap of ADHD with conduct problems in childhood results from a common set of genetic factors, but that the development of conduct problems is also influenced by the familial environment. Recent data found that certain alleles of the catechol-0-methyl transferase gene increase risk for conduct problems in children with ADHD [16]. The combination of ADHD and conduct problems has been found to be a familial subtype of ADHD in the sense that they are found to aggregate together within close family members.

Prevention strategies are thought to be important to protect vulnerable children with ADHD from exposure to detrimental environments that increase the risk for conduct problems. These may include difficulty in developing secure parent child attachments, inconsistent or abusive parenting, and exposure to negative peer influences. This may be particularly important if a child with ADHD has difficulties in forming healthy social relationships and has problems at school, including exclusion.

The interplay between genetic and environmental factors in the development of comorbidities is undoubtedly complex and the subject of much ongoing research, but there is a clear implication that ADHD should be detected early so that strategies can be put in place to prevent the development of co-occurring behavioral problems later in life.

Drug abuse

Developmental pathways from ADHD into drug abuse and addiction are multi-faceted and include three main components: impulsive risk-taking behavior, use of drugs to reduce ADHD symptoms (self-medication), and the consequences of increased exposure and sensitivity to environonmental risks factors.

ADHD is associated with impulsive risk taking behaviors which form an inherent component of the disorder. This may relate to deficits in reward processing that have been identified in ADHD [17,18] and a relatively large improvement in performance when task performance is linked to rewards [19]. It may also be the case that the distorted perception associated with some substances may be particularly appealing to individuals who are highly sensation-seeking.

Another likely explanation is that many adults with ADHD self-medicate with substances such as cannabis and alcohol to reduce symptoms such as ceaseless mental processes, restlessness, and difficulty falling asleep [20–22]. Some describe using stimulant drugs such as cocaine and amphetamines and experiencing a paradoxical calming effect associated with reduction of ADHD symptoms [23], although this appears to be less common than the use of either alcohol or cannabis.

ADHD may also be associated with a lifelong history of impairments and exposure to detrimental psychosocial environments that can lead to an increased risk of addiction [24]. Addiction may also develop as one of the consequences of comorbid conduct disorder. It has been reported that drug abuse is initiated an average of 3 years earlier in ADHD compared to non-ADHD cases, which is important because early age of drug use is linked to the development of substance use disorders, and individuals with ADHD are more likely to progress from an alcohol-use disorder to a drug-use disorder [24]. The relatively high rates of ADHD within drug abuse populations had led to concerns that the use of prescribed stimulants to treat ADHD might lead to addiction problems. However, follow-up studies of stimulant-treated and untreated groups of children with ADHD found no increase in rates of drug abuse problems [25]. In fact, there is some evidence of a reduction back towards general population rates [26].

Diagnosis and treatment of attention deficit hyperactivity disorder and comorbid disorders

Mood disorders

Problems with mood instability, emotional over-reactivity, and temper outbursts are commonly seen in adults with ADHD and in some cases are the main presenting complaints [4,6]. Clinical experience, supported by clinical trials [9,10], shows that mood instability in adults with ADHD usually responds to stimulant medication and atomoxetine in the same time course as the main ADHD symptoms, and should therefore be regarded as part of the ADHD condition, and not always reflecting a separate mood disorder. Careful evaluation will need to be made of any affective symptoms, to differentiate the mood lability associated with ADHD from anxiety, depression, bipolar, and personality disorders (Table 6.1).

Attention deficit hyperactivity disorder and bipolar disorder

The frequency of comorbid bipolar disorder and ADHD continues to be hotly contested [7]. The crux of the debate centers on the presentation of ADHD symptoms alongside chronic irritability, aggression, and mood lability and whether this represents ADHD, bipolar disorder, their co-occurrence, or a distinct psychiatric disorder. This is a particular concern in child and adolescent psychiatry, where modified criteria for 'juvenile bipolar disorder' overlap with those for 'severe mood dysregulation.' However, it is also the case that ADHD in adults

Key clinical characteristics that distinguish between attention deficit hyperactivity disorder, bipolar disorder, and borderline personality disorders

	Borderline	Bipolar
Similarities with ADHD	• Childhood or adolescent onset • Developmentally inappropriate behaviors • Chronic trait like course • Pervasive across situations • Impulsivity • Impaired social relationships • Emotional/mood instability • Irritability	• Overactivity • Pressured/incessant speech • Impulsivity • Irritability • Emotional/mood instability • Distractibility • Short attention span • Depressive episodes (not uncommon in ADHD) • Sleep problems
Differences from ADHD	• Frantic efforts to avoid real or imagined abandonment • Identify disturbance • Recurrent suicidal behaviour • Chronic feelings of emptiness • Transient stress-related paranoid thoughts	• Episodic course • Post-pubertal onset • Grandiose or elated mood • Often lacks insight • Psychosis
ADHD specific symptoms	• Inattention • Overactivity	• Trait-like course • Early childhood onset • Insight

Table 6.1 Key clinical characteristics that distinguish between attention deficit hyperactivity disorder, bipolar disorder, and borderline personality disorders.

is sometimes misdiagnosed as bipolar disorder. This is clearly important for patients since the incorrect treatment can lead to nonresponse, unnecessary side effects, and the exacerbation of symptoms.

In clinical practice, this problem arises particularly in relation to broader definitions of bipolar disorder, including bipolar II (when the episodic criteria are ignored, or mood instability is considered a form or ultra-rapid cycling) and cyclothymia. Overlapping symptoms include overactive behavior, physical restlessness, mood changes, irritability, aggression, and distractibility. However, the temporal qualities of the presenting symptoms should differentiate between the two disorders in most cases. ADHD is a trait-like condition arising in childhood, with associated chronicity of symptoms and impairments. By comparison, DSM-IV characterizes mania as a 'distinct period' of abnormal mood, indicating that this occurs during a discrete period of time, where there is a change from the premorbid state and the onset of new symptoms [13]. The differences can be summarized in the following way: in ADHD, symptoms are abnormal in relation to developmental norms, whereas in bipolar disorder, symptoms are abnormal in relation to the premorbid mental state.

The distinction therefore requires a detailed enquiry into the mental state of the person, and careful account needs to be taken of the onset and developmental course of co-occurring mood symptoms. Compared to bipolar disorder, ADHD has a much earlier age of onset and a chronic, persistent course. Mood swings are less extreme and more frequent (around four or five times a day), are interspersed by short periods of normal mood, and there are no extended periods of very low or high moods. Grandiosity is not a feature of ADHD. Thoughts may be ceaseless and unfocused (a distracted mind) but are not speeded up, do not show flight of ideas, and are not experienced as unusually clear or special. In some cases, differential diagnosis may be difficult, particularly when ADHD symptoms are severe, and it is possible to have both conditions.

Attention deficit hyperactivity disorder and depression

People with ADHD are more likely to suffer depressive episodes than non-ADHD controls [27]. However, a common problem in ADHD is chronic low self esteem and dysthymia, which in the presence of concentration difficulties may lead to a misdiagnosis of depression as the primary disorder [28,29]. Furthermore, some of the symptoms of ADHD may overlap with those found in depression. These include sleep problems, restlessness or agitation, apathy and lack of motivation, lack of interest in usual daily activities, and in some cases, low levels of energy for anything that is not immediately rewarding [30].

The distinction between ADHD and depression is usually made by attention to the early onset and chronic course of symptoms associated with ADHD, whereas a depressive episode is usually identified by a change from the usual premorbid mental state. Symptoms related closely to ADHD usually persist in a chronic trait-like way and would be present during euthymic, as well as dysthymic, periods.

Treatment of attention deficit hyperactivity disorder and mood disorders

The following are recommendations from UKAAN for treating comorbid ADHD with a mood disorder:

- An irritable or unstable mood is frequently seen in adults with ADHD and is not usually the consequence of comorbid depression or bipolar disorder. In this case, treatment should be targeted at ADHD.
- Mood instability may also arise as part of a major affective disorder and care must therefore be taken to ensure that mood lability does not occur solely within the context of a depressive or manic/hypomanic episode. This is determined predominantly by attending to the time course of the symptoms (ie, early onset, chronic trait-like course, frequency of mood swings), and the detailed psychopathology (ie, whether the mood swings are extreme, sustained for longer periods, or are associated with other features of major affective disorder). Where there is a clear cyclical mood disorder, treatment with mood stabilizers or antidepressants usually takes priority over other treatments.
- Some individuals previously diagnosed with atypical depression, cyclothymia, or emotionally unstable personality disorder (who may or may not also fulfill criteria for these diagnoses) will have a primary diagnosis of ADHD with good response to stimulants. A previous history of such diagnoses should therefore not exclude the possibility of ADHD as the primary diagnosis.
- Individuals with ADHD may present with an episode of depression that requires treatment. In this case, treatment of depression would usually be the priority because of the risks of untreated depression. Moreover, persistence of major depression may interfere with the efficacy of treatments for ADHD. Patients who are effectively treated for ADHD may report a 'falling off' of the beneficial effects of stimulant treatment and experience a return of ADHD symptoms during episodes of depression.

- The severity of ADHD symptoms and the need for stimulant medication can be re-evaluated once the comorbid depression has been treated.
- If the depression is of relatively recent onset and is not too severe (in adults with untreated ADHD), it may be worth considering a brief trial of stimulants before long-term treatment with antidepressants.
- Data on the combined use of antidepressants and stimulants are lacking. Clinical experience suggests that the combination of antidepressants with stimulants could be particularly important where the persistence of ADHD symptoms is thought to contribute to the maintenance depression. This may occur if, for example, persistent problems with ADHD symptoms cause difficulties with self-organization or personal relationships, leading to high levels of stress.

Figure 6.1 depicts an algorithm for treating adults with mood instability.

Substance abuse and addiction

Substance use and addiction disorders are relatively common comorbid conditions when compared to rates in the non-ADHD population. Most studies of ADHD estimate rates of all types of substance abuse use to be around twice the population rate, and among addiction clinic populations 10% or more are found to have a current full diagnosis of ADHD [31]. As discussed, the causes of the relationship are complex and individuals with ADHD who do not receive sufficient treatment during childhood are thought to be at particular risk of developing substance abuse and addiction problems later in life.

The most common forms of drug misuse in ADHD are alcohol and cannabis [20–22]. These are widely available, and patients with ADHD symptoms often describe using one or other of these to help reduce symptoms such as mental and physical restlessness, and in order to help them relax. The use of these drugs is not always at a harmful level but regular use of any drug is of potential concern.

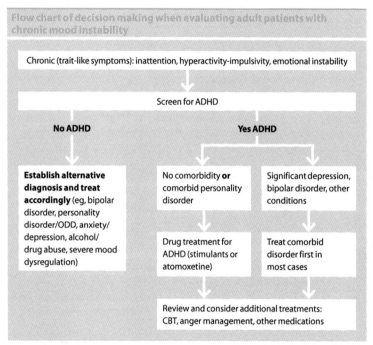

Figure 6.1 Flow chart of decision making when evaluating adult patients with chronic mood instability. ADHD, attention deficit hyperactivity disorder; CBT, cognitive behavioral therapy; ODD, oppositional defiant disorder.

More serious use of alcohol, cannabis, amphetamine, cocaine, or opiates are also seen among individuals with ADHD. In recent (as yet unpublished) surveys in South London and across Europe, rates of ADHD averaged around 10–12% in patients attending addiction detoxification units; yet very few of these patients had been diagnosed or treated for ADHD either as children or adults.

Treatment of attention deficit hyperactivity disorder and substance abuse disorders

The potential benefits of treating ADHD in individuals with substance use disorders are considerable, although there are few formal evaluations in the literature [32]. ADHD is not only associated with increased risk of alcohol and drug addiction, but is also thought to be associated with nonsubstance related addictive behaviors such as pathological gambling and internet addiction [33,34]. So far, it remains unclear how far treatment will counteract such behaviors. However, it seems likely that timely and sufficient ADHD treatment with adequate psychosocial support can help to treat addictions or at least reduce their severity.

The likely outcome of treating ADHD depends on the type and nature of the drug abuse or addiction and the overall level of function of the individual. The potential benefits from better control and reduction of ADHD symptoms include the following:

- increased level of function, enabling the person to focus on work and other useful activities;
- increased level of interest in daily activities and reduced need for risk-taking behaviors, including drug taking;
- reduced need to self-medicate to control ADHD symptoms;
- increased ability to attend and focus on, and therefore, benefit from individual or group therapy sessions;
- increased resilience and the ability to cope with failures without resorting to alcohol or drug use.

Service delivery issues

Whether an individual with a drug or alcohol problem can take advantage of these potential benefits depends on both individual factors (including personality traits such as novelty seeking), the reason for the substance abuse and the substance in question. One common stumbling block is lack of engagement and commitment to the treatment process. Poor compliance with clinical assessments, treatments, and follow-up is a major hindrance for the successful treatment of ADHD, as well as the abuse or addiction disorder. Positive outcomes are more likely for those who recognize and acknowledge their problems and the need for treatment.

Treatment is therefore best delivered by close liaison between specialist ADHD and substance misuse services. Ideally, treatment for ADHD would be delivered by drug and alcohol teams who are trained in the recognition and treatment of ADHD, but in practice it often requires joint cooperation between specialist ADHD and addiction teams.

Treatment choice

The treatment of choice for adults with ADHD is stimulant medication. However, concerns exist about their use in patients in substance use disorders. The main risks are:

- poor compliance (not taking prescribed medication);
- diversion (giving away or selling drugs to other people);
- abuse (taking nonprescribed stimulants or injecting or snorting stimulants).

In practice, there is limited evidence for abuse, but high rates of diversion, particularly among college students to help in their studies, have been reported in the US [35]. Compliance with treatment regimes, particularly with short-acting medication that has to be taken several times a day, can also be a challenge.

Risk of abuse and potential for addiction to attention deficit hyperactivity disorder medications

The risk of abuse of methylphenidate has been investigated and has been shown to be related to the mode of delivery of the drug [36,37]. Methylphenidate increases extracellular dopamine in the brain, which has both reinforcing and therapeutic effects. Abuse potential occurs when the drug effect is perceived as particularly salient to the individual. This was found to be related to several factors including important pharmacokinetic effects, rapid changes in serum concentrations, and subsequent rapid dopamine increases (as is achieved with intravenous injection). This is akin to a burst-like 'phasic' release pattern of dopamine.

Conversely, the therapeutic effects are associated with slowly ascending serum concentrations and smoothly rising dopamine levels (as is achieved with oral administration). The slow, steady-state, dopamine increases mimic those of the brains tonic firing (or smooth) release pattern. Should there be doubts either about a patient's compliance or, potential for abuse or diversion, there are two main treatment choices:

- use atomoxetine as drug of choice (low abuse and diversion potential, dosing can be once-daily);
- use long-acting formulations of methylphenidate or pro-drugs that have a relatively slow uptake of the active stimulant

(low abuse and diversion potential, once-daily dosing). The two main choices are:

- Concerta® XL: due to the delivery system, methylphenidate capsules are difficult to extract for injection or intranasal administration (see Chapter 7).
- Vyvanse®: a pro-drug of dexamphetamine that is inactive until ingested (or injected), has relatively slow uptake of active drug into the brain and therefore has low abuse potential (see Chapter 7).

Does the use of stimulants increase the risk of addiction?

There are several studies suggesting that early treatment of ADHD may prevent substance use disorder in later life, and certainly does not increase the risk of later addiction [38]. Furthermore, children and adolescents with ADHD who are prescribed stimulant medication to control ADHD symptoms do not develop addiction to their medication. Indeed, during adolescence, compliance with drug treatments for ADHD is a problem, even in those who have been on medication for a long time.

Anxiety disorders and attention deficit hyperactivity disorder

ADHD in adults is frequently associated with anxiety disorders. Social phobia is particularly frequent with prevalence estimates as high as 20–34% in some studies [39]. ADHD is more frequent in adult patients with panic disorder than in controls and the associated functional impairments also tend to be greater [40]. Though few studies have been conducted in this area, there is evidence that the presence of a comorbid anxiety disorder is associated with more pronounced attentional deficits and with a higher susceptibility to drug and alcohol abuse [38].

Differentiation of anxiety disorders in attention deficit hyperactivity disorder

Individuals should always be screened for symptoms of anxiety disorders whenever ADHD is being evaluated. Particular attention should be paid to the onset and course of symptoms because anxiety itself may be associated with attention problems and anxious ruminations that mimic the attentional deficits in ADHD. Somatic symptoms and the presence of panic attacks make the distinction from ADHD clear.

Treatment of anxiety disorders in attention deficit hyperactivity disorder

UKAAN recommends that, in general, treatment of anxiety disorders should be offered in conjunction with ADHD treatment. Selective serotonin reuptake inhibitors (SSRIs) are effective in anxiety disorders and should usually be used as the first-line drug treatment [41]. There are, however, specific considerations when evaluating anxiety states in ADHD:

- People with ADHD are likely to have some level of anxiety as a normal response to problems related to the symptoms and impairments of ADHD. For individuals where the anxiety disorder is generalized and not too severe, treating ADHD first is often the best strategy [42].
- Stimulants can trigger panic attacks or worsen somatic anxiety in some people, particularly in those with a previous history of somatic anxiety. In such cases, consider initiating an SSRI or other anti-anxiety agent at the same time as starting stimulants [41]. Atomoxetine is a useful option as it does not have the potential anxiogenic effects of stimulants [42].
- Where there is a clearly identifiable anxiety disorder, this would usually be treated before the ADHD is addressed. The level of ADHD symptoms can then be re-evaluated once there is better control of the anxiety. Treatment of the anxiety may include medication and psychotherapeutic interventions such as cognitive behavioral therapy (CBT) [41]. However, underlying ADHD symptoms may play a role in maintaining the anxiety symptoms or may hinder engagement with CBT, in which case it may be important to initiate treatment for ADHD at the same time.
- Methylphenidate has been demonstrated to reduce trait anxiety in some children [43] and may have a similar effect in young adults. Whether atomoxetine is of specific benefit in the presence of comorbid anxiety is still unclear. Some studies point to an effect

on social phobia [44], while others have not found any particular benefit when ADHD is comorbid with anxiety disorders [45].

Attention deficit hyperactivity disorder and obsessive compulsive disorder

In contrast to other anxiety disorders, adults with ADHD do not have an excess lifetime prevalence of obsessive compulsive disorder (OCD) [39,40,43–46]. However, studies conducted in children and adolescents present an entirely different picture. Up to 11% of children with ADHD fulfill the criteria for OCD, and 30% of adolescents with OCD also have ADHD [47]. This is far in excess of prevalence estimates for OCD of 2.8–4.5% in children and 0.3–4.0% in adolescents [48]. There is some evidence that ADHD and pediatric OCD may cosegregate, suggesting that this combination may be a specific familial subtype of ADHD [49].

From a clinical perspective, children with both ADHD and OCD are thought to have more psychosocial impairment than those with only one diagnosis; whether the same is true in adults remains unclear. It has been suggested that adults with ADHD may use repetitive, almost compulsive, routines as a coping mechanism to compensate for attentional symptoms and the experience of recurrent forgetfulness. Following a strict, predetermined order while doing common tasks like cooking or driving can be understood as a compensatory strategy to minimize impairment. These behaviors may reduce or disappear once the patient is successfully treated for ADHD. When strict routines and repetitive patterns of behaviors are found as core symptoms, the possibility of comorbid Asperger's syndrome should be considered.

Diagnosis

Exploration of OCD symptoms is particularly relevant in young adults. In most cases, the comorbidity is diagnosed by evaluation of the mental state with close attention to descriptions of any obsessions and compulsions. Diagnostic considerations specific to ADHD includes the following:

- The repetitive thought processes that characterize OCD may be difficult to distinguish from ceaseless and distractible thought processes often seen in adults with ADHD.

- Excessive mental activity or the feeling of being always 'on the go' is common in ADHD. Adults with ADHD often report a continuous stream of thoughts that prevent them both from concentrating on tasks and may be described as 'exhausting.' These thoughts are not, however, usually experienced as intrusive or repetitive and should not be classified as obsessive ruminations.
- When both pathologies coexist, related problems such as tics or ASD may also be present.
- Some people with ADHD adopt strict routines and may repeatedly check that they have completed tasks or not forgotten something to cope with ADHD symptoms such as disorganization and forgetfulness. They may also become anxious when such routines are interrupted. Careful attention to the reasons for their behavior and their relationship to either ADHD symptoms or obsessions should enable distinction of the two disorders in most cases.

Treatment

Further studies in adults are needed to clarify the optimal treatment approach in the case of comorbidity between ADHD and OCD. It is advised to treat both conditions separately in order to maximize therapeutic response. In general, pharmacological treatment for OCD will include an SSRI at a high dose. Clomipramine is also effective, but the risk of adverse events is higher [50]. Comorbid ADHD should be treated using standard approaches.

References

1 Kessler RC, Green JG, Adler LA, et al. Structure and diagnosis of adult attention-deficit/hyperactivity disorder: analysis of expanded symptom criteria from the Adult ADHD clinical diagnostic scale. *Arch General Psych.* 2010;67:1168-1178.
2 Barkley R, Murphy KR, Fischer M. *ADHD in Adults: What the Science Says.* New York: Guilford Press; 2007.
3 Brown TE. Executive functions and attention deficit hyperactivity disorder: Implications of two conflicting views. *Int J Disabil Dev Edu.* 2006;53:35-46.
4 Asherson P. Clinical assessment and treatment of attention deficit hyperactivity disorder in adults. *Expert Rev Neurother.* 2005;5:525-539.
5 Barkley RA, Fischer M. The unique contribution of emotional impulsiveness to impairment in major life activities in hyperactive children as adults. *J Am Acad Child Adolesc Psychiatry.* 2010;49:503-513.

6   Skirrow C, McLoughlin G, Kuntsi J, Asherson P. Behavioral, neurocognitive and treatment overlap between attention-deficit/hyperactivity disorder and mood instability. *Expert Rev Neurother.* 2009;9:489-503.

7   Skirrow C, Hosang GM, Farmer AE, Asherson P. An update on the debated association between ADHD and bipolar disorder across the lifespan. *J Affect Disord.* 2012.

8   Reimherr FW, Marchant BK, Strong RE, et al. Emotional dysregulation in adult ADHD and response to atomoxetine. *Biol Psych.* 2005;58:125-131.

9   Reimherr FW, Williams ED, Strong RE, Mestas R, Soni P, Marchant BK. A double-blind, placebo-controlled, crossover study of osmotic release oral system methylphenidate in adults with ADHD with assessment of oppositional and emotional dimensions of the disorder. *J Clin Psychiatry.* 2007;68:93-101.

10 Rosler M, Retz W, Fischer R, et al. Twenty-four-week treatment with extended release methylphenidate improves emotional symptoms in adult ADHD. *World J Biol Psych.* 2010;11:709-718.

11 Kuntsi J, Eley TC, Taylor A, et al. Co-occurrence of ADHD and low IQ has genetic origins. *Am J Med Genet B Neuropsychiatr Genet.* 2004;124B:41-47.

12 National Institute for Health and Clinical Excellence. Attention Deficit Hyperactivity Disorder: the NICE Guideline on Diagnosis and Managment of ADHD in Children, Young People and Adults. Clinical Guidelines, CG72. NICE website. www.nice.org.uk/CG72. Accessed August 25, 2012.

13 American Psychiatry Association (APA). *Diagnostic and Statistical Manual of Mental Disorders.* 4th edition, text revision. Washington DC: American Psychiatric Association; 2000.

14 Willcutt EG, Pennington BF, Olson RK, DeFries JC. Understanding comorbidity: a twin study of reading disability and attention-deficit/hyperactivity disorder. *Am J Med Genet B Neuropsychiatr Genet.* 2007;144B:709-714.

15 Ronald A, Simonoff E, Kuntsi J, Asherson P, Plomin R. Evidence for overlapping genetic influences on autistic and ADHD behaviours in a community twin sample. *J Child Psychol Psychiatry.* 2008;49:535-542.

16 Caspi A, Langley K, Milne B, et al. A replicated molecular genetic basis for subtyping antisocial behavior in children with attention-deficit/hyperactivity disorder. *Arch Gen Psychiatry.* 2008;65:203-210.

17 Scheres A, Milham MP, Knutson B, Castellanos FX. Ventral striatal hyporesponsiveness during reward anticipation in attention-deficit/hyperactivity disorder. *Biol Psych.* 2007;61:720-724.

18 Paloyelis Y, Asherson P, Mehta MA, Faraone SV, Kuntsi J. DAT1 and COMT effects on delay discounting and trait impulsivity in male adolescents with attention deficit/hyperactivity disorder and healthy controls. *Neuropsychopharmacology.* 2010;35:2414-2426.

19 Andreou P, Neale BM, Chen W, et al. Reaction time performance in ADHD: improvement under fast-incentive condition and familial effects. *Psychol Med.* 2007;37:1703-1715.

20 Wilson JJ, Levin FR. Attention deficit hyperactivity disorder (ADHD) and substance use disorders. *Curr Psychiatry Rep.* 2001;3:497-506.

21 Biederman J, Wilens T, Mick E, Milberger S, Spencer TJ, Faraone SV. Psychoactive substance use disorders in adults with attention deficit hyperactivity disorder (ADHD): effects of ADHD and psychiatric comorbidity. *Am J Psychiatry.* 1995; 152: 1652-1658.

22 Ohlmeier MD, Peters K, Te Wildt BT, Zedler M, Ziegenbein M, Wiese B, et al. Comorbidity of alcohol and substance dependence with attention-deficit/hyperactivity disorder (ADHD). *Alcohol Alcohol.* 2008; 43: 300-304.

23 Lambert N. The contribution of childhood ADHD, conduct problems, and stimulant treatment to adolescent and adult tobacco and psychoactive substance abuse. *Ethical Hum Psychol Psychiatry.* 2005;7:197-221.

24 Wilens TE, Kwon A, Tanguay S, et al. Characteristics of adults with attention deficit hyperactivity disorder plus substance use disorder: the role of psychiatric comorbidity. *Am J Addict.* 2005;14:319-327.

25 Nelson A, Galon P. Exploring the relationship among ADHD, stimulants, and substance abuse. *J Child Adolesc Psychiatr Nurs*. 2012;25:113-118.

26 Wilens TE, Faraone SV, Biederman J, Gunawardene S. Does stimulant therapy of attention-deficit/hyperactivity disorder beget later substance abuse? A meta-analytic review of the literature. *Pediatrics*. 2003;111:179-185.

27 Meinzer MC, Pettit JW, Leventhal AM, Hill RM. Explaining the covariance between attention-deficit hyperactivity disorder symptoms and depressive symptoms: the role of hedonic responsivity. *J Clin Psychol*. 2012;[Epub ahead of print].

28 Edbom T, Lichtenstein P, Granlund M, Larsson JO. Long-term relationships between symptoms of attention deficit hyperactivity disorder and self-esteem in a prospective longitudinal study of twins. *Acta Paediatr*. 2006;95:650-657.

29 Shekim WO, Asarnow RF, Hess E, Zaucha K, Wheeler N. A clinical and demographic profile of a sample of adults with attention deficit hyperactivity disorder, residual state. *Compr Psychiatry*. 1990;31:416-425.

30 Doyle BD. *Understanding and Treating Adults with Attention Deficit Hyperactivity Disorder*. Washington DC, American Psychiatric Publishing; 2006.

31 Kessler RC, Adler L, Barkley R, et al. The prevalence and correlates of adult ADHD in the United States: results from the National Comorbidity Survey Replication. *Am J Psychiatry*. 2006;163:716-723.

32 Magon R, Müller U. ADHD with comorbid substance use disorder: review of treatment. *Adv Psychiatr*. 2012;18:436-446.

33 Yen JY, Yen CF, Chen CS, Tang TC, Ko CH. The association between adult ADHD symptoms and internet addiction among college students: the gender difference. *Cyberpsychol Behav*. 2009;12:187-191.

34 Breyer JL, Botzet AM, Winters KC, Stinchfield RD, August G, Realmuto G. Young adult gambling behaviors and their relationship with the persistence of ADHD. *J Gambl Stud*. 2009;25:227-238.

35 Wilens TE, Adler LA, Adams J, et al. Misuse and diversion of stimulants prescribed for ADHD: a systematic review of the literature. *J Am Acad Child Adolesc Psychiatry*. 2008;47:21-31.

36 Volkow ND, Swanson JM. Variables that affect the clinical use and abuse of methylphenidate in the treatment of ADHD. *Am J Psychiatry*. 2003;160:1909-1918.

37 Swanson JM, Volkow ND. Serum and brain concentrations of methylphenidate: implications for use and abuse. *Neurosci Biobehav Rev*. 2003;27:615-621.

38 Faraone SV, Wilens T. Does stimulant treatment lead to substance use disorders? *J Clin Psychiatry*. 2003;64(suppl 11):9-13.

39 Sobanski E. Psychiatric comorbidity in adults with attention-deficit/hyperactivity disorder (ADHD). *Eur Arch Psychiatry Clin Neurosci*. 2006;256(suppl 1):i26-i31.

40 Fones CS, Pollack MH, Susswein L, Otto M. History of childhood attention deficit hyperactivity disorder (ADHD) features among adults with panic disorder. *J Affect Disord*. 2000;58:99-106.

41 Dodson WW. Pharmacotherapy of adult ADHD. *J Clin Psychol*. 2005;61:589-606.

42 41. Asherson P. Clinical assessment and treatment of attention deficit hyperactivity disorder in adults. *Expert Rev Neurotherapeutics*. 2005;5:525-539.

43 Gurkan K, Bilgic A, Turkoglu S, Kilic BG, Aysev A, Uslu R. Depression, anxiety and obsessive-compulsive symptoms and quality of life in children with attention-deficit hyperactivity disorder (ADHD) during three-month methylphenidate treatment. *J Psychopharmacol*. 2010;24:1810-1818.

44 Adler LA, Liebowitz M, Kronenberger W, et al. Atomoxetine treatment in adults with attention-deficit/hyperactivity disorder and comorbid social anxiety disorder. *Depress Anxiety*. 2009;26:212-221.

45 Scott NG, Ripperger-Suhler J, Rajab MH, Kjar D. Factors associated with atomoxetine efficacy for treatment of attention-deficit/hyperactivity disorder in children and adolescents. *J Child Adolesc Psychopharmacol*. 2010;20:197-203.

46 Babcock T, Ornstein CS. Comorbidity and its impact in adult patients with attention-deficit/hyperactivity disorder: a primary care perspective. *Postgrad Med.* 2009;121:73-82.

47 Geller DA, Biederman J, Faraone SV, et al. Attention-deficit/hyperactivity disorder in children and adolescents with obsessive-compulsive disorder: fact or artifact? *J Am Acad Child Adolesc Psychiatry.* 2002;41:52-58.

48 Fogel J. An epidemiological perspective of obsessive-compulsive disorder in children and adolescents. *Can Child Adolesc Psychiatr Rev.* 2003;12:33-36.

49 Geller D, Petty C, Vivas F, Johnson J, Pauls D, Biederman J. Further evidence for co-segregation between pediatric obsessive compulsive disorder and attention deficit hyperactivity disorder: a familial risk analysis. *Biol Psych.* 2007;61:1388-1394.

50 Bandelow B. The medical treatment of obsessive-compulsive disorder and anxiety. *CNS Spectr.* 2008;13(9 suppl 14):37-46.

Chapter 7

Pharmacological treatments

Choice of drug therapy

Drug treatment is the recommended first-line treatment for attention deficit hyperactivity disorder (ADHD) in adults. There are two main classes of drugs available [1–3]:

- stimulants (eg, methylphenidate, dexamphetamine, modafinil);
- nonstimulants (eg, atomoxetine, bupropion, clonidine, tricyclic antidepressants, venlafaxine).

In Europe, the stimulant methylphenidate is recommended as the drug of choice, with dexamphetamine as an excellent alternative option [4]. The main reason for this distinction is the availability of a wider range of short-acting and long-acting formulations for methylphenidate and the perception of a greater abuse potential for dexamphetamine (although this has not been proven).

The non-stimulant atomoxetine is usually considered a second-line treatment mainly because of its slightly lower efficacy in drug trials and its slower onset of beneficial effects when compared with the stimulants [5]. However, atomoxetine has particular benefits because of its lack of abuse or diversion potential and because the effects are stable with once- or twice-daily dosing [6].

Bupropion, modafinil, clonidine, tricyclic antidepressants, and venlafaxine have also proved beneficial in clinical trials but their effect sizes are significantly smaller than that of methylphenidate and there are far fewer clinical trials evaluating efficacy in ADHD. They are therefore

UKAAN, *Handbook for Attention Deficit Hyperactivity Disorder in Adults*, DOI: 10.1007/978-1-908517-79-1_7, © Springer Healthcare 2013

recommended by the National Institute for Health and Clinical Excellence (NICE) as third-line agents [1].

At the time of publication, in the UK, methylphenidate, dexamphetamine, and atomoxetine are currently licensed for first time use in children and adolescents but not for adults. However, atomoxetine is licensed for continued use in adults when started before the age of 18 years and Concerta (a long acting formulation of methylphenidate) when the person received the diagnosis of ADHD and treatment before the age of 18 years. Therefore, the prescription of ADHD medication in adults is often off-label.

However, there is sufficient scientific evidence, which is well documented in the literature, that both stimulants and atomoxetine are effective and safe when used to treat ADHD in adults [7–10]. Guidance for clinicians in the UK on the off-label use of these medications for the treatment of ADHD is provided by National Institute for Health and Clinical Excellence (NICE) [1] and other professional bodies (eg, British Association for Psychopharmacology) [2,4].

According to the NICE guidelines, stimulant treatment should be considered the first-line therapy for the management of ADHD in adults [1]. The guidelines recommend the use of methylphenidate as first-line treatment choice, except when there is a risk of abuse or diversion. In this situation, atomoxetine is preferred. When there is no improvement (over a 6-week trial period) or there are intolerable side effects with methylphenidate, either atomoxetine or dexamphetamine should be considered. Extended-release (ER) preparations of methylphenidate may provide sufficient control of ADHD symptoms with only a single daily dose taken in the morning [1]. The NICE guidelines do not offer advice on which drugs should be considered for third-line use, but based on expert opinion we recommend the use of buproprion (see Figure 7.1).

The prescription of any medications for ADHD should be part of a comprehensive treatment program that addresses psychological, behavioral, educational, or occupational needs, including the use of psychological treatments. The choice of drug should take into account comorbid conditions, differing adverse effects, potential for drug misuse, and the preferences of the patient and carers [1].

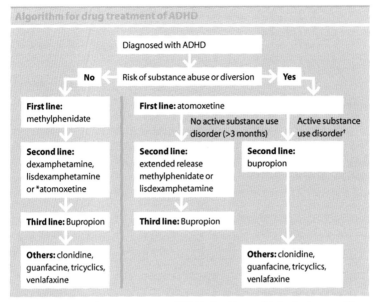

Figure 7.1 Algorithm for drug treatment of ADHD. *Consider possible first line in cases with comorbid anxiety with panic attacks; †Potential for abuse of stimulants needs to be evaluated. Stimulants may be used in some cases of cannabis or alcohol use disorders, depending on evaluation of compliance and potential for abuse of stimulants.

Drug prescribing

Drug treatment for adults with ADHD should be initiated by a psychiatrist or another clinical prescriber with experience in the management and treatment of ADHD. NICE guidance on the general principles of prescribing is summarized in Table 7.1 [1]. Where there is adequate supervision from a specialist with experience in the management and treatment of ADHD and, ideally, there are shared care agreements in place, prescriptions can be initiated by primary care. During the maintenance phase of treatment, routine prescribing, and physical health checks are usually provided by primary care with at least annual specialist review, again ideally under a shared care protocol.

Drug monitoring

Once medication for ADHD is initiated, it is important that there is appropriate monitoring. NICE recommends that a drug-monitoring service

General principles for prescribing drugs for adults with attention deficit hyperactivity disorder

- Prescribers should be familiar with pharmacokinetic profiles of all available preparations to ensure treatment is tailored to individual needs
- Prescribers should be familiar with controlled drug legislation
- Dosages of stimulants should be increased until there is no further clinical improvement, and side effects remain tolerable
- Following titration and dose stabilization, prescribing should be carried out under locally agreed shared care agreements with primary care
- Side effects should be routinely monitored and documented
- Treatment should be reviewed at least annually

Table 7.1 General principles for prescribing drugs for adults with attention deficit hyperactivity disorder. Adapted from NICE [1].

be established and provided by suitably trained specialists, including nurse practitioners [1]. The aim of such a service is to:

- monitor initial response to medication;
- provide guidance on titration and dosage;
- monitor for adverse effects;
- review ongoing effects and continued need for medication.

The response to medication is primarily evaluated by comparing symptom control against side effects. During the titration phase, symptoms and side effects should be recorded at each review. Feedback should be sought, wherever possible, from an informant such as a spouse, parent, or close friend. Initial follow-up can be provided face to face or by telephone, depending on the medication prescribed, the reliability of the patient, and the experience of the prescriber. Certain cases, for example, a patient who has been on ADHD medication in the past, may require less rigorous follow-up by a specialist service.

Drug titration and treatment response

Gradual titration is required when using stimulants in order to achieve optimal control of symptoms. The aims of the titration process for stimulants are:

- to adapt the dosage to the highly variable individual response;
- to balance the symptomatic response against side effects and risks.

During the titration phase, doses should be progressively increased in a cautious stepwise fashion until there is no further clinical improvement (ie, reduction in symptoms, beneficial behavior change, and improved function in education, employment, and relationships) and side effects remain tolerable [1]. Some useful tips to guide the titration process are listed in Table 7.2.

For each patient it is important to establish the specific symptoms that they wish to target and individual aims for treatment; bearing in mind that the patient's definition of symptom control may differ from the prescriber's. It is therefore essential to get clear feedback from the patient and allow them to guide the titration process. The ideal dose may not always be the one that gives complete control of symptoms. Not every patient is happy with the effect of the medication on their symptoms and some may report feeling overmedicated, especially if the dose is too high. Typical descriptions indicating the need to consider lowering the dose or changing the medication include:

- "the medication is too controlling;"
- "I'm just not 'me' anymore;"
- "my head feels empty;"
- loss of spontaneity or quickness of thought;
- loss of creativity;
- loss of social appeal (ie, "I used to be the life and soul of the party and now I feel that I'm just boring");
- the feeling of having undergone a period of adjustment and a fundamental change in personality.

Although many people are able to verbalize their response to treatment when asked open questions, some find it more difficult. Diaries or charts

Useful tips for titrating stimulants

- Titrate the dose against symptoms and side effects over a 4- to 10-week period
- Titrate slowly if there is a history of tics or seizures
- If side effects become troublesome, consider a dose reduction
- If patient is not tolerating treatment, consider using alternative formulations or alternative medications
- Manage the patient's expectations
- Consider follow-up via telephone (if appropriate)
- Arrange weekly, fortnightly, or monthly follow-up
- Record symptoms and side effects at each review
- Where possible, get collateral feedback (eg, from a spouse, parent, or close friend)

Table 7.2 Useful tips for titrating stimulants.

can be used to plot symptoms and side effects. These can serve as a prompt during clinical reviews.

To ensure a systematic approach, at various stages during the titration period symptom levels can be measured using rating scales. These are typically the same questionnaires used for screening. Side-effect and impairment scales also exist and can be of benefit (see Appendix J). Some patients have difficulty noticing any effects from medication, when reports from those around them, such as a spouse or colleague, indicate that their presentation has improved, often quite markedly. During the titration period, standard questions at each review could include:

- *What dose are you currently taking?* This may vary from the prescribed dose due to patient error. For example, patients may get used to taking a certain number of tablets and not realize the tablet strength has increased with a new prescription. Prescribers may also mistakenly prescribe a different formulation (eg, extended-release instead of instant-release), especially if they are unfamiliar with the medications.

- *When do you take the medication and how long do the effects last?* When exactly are the dosages taken, after how long does the patient begin to notice the effects and when do the effects start wearing off.

- *What effects does the medication have?* The identification at assessment of key symptoms that the patient wishes to target may help to focus the titration phase of treatment, making it easier for the patient and health care professional to identify specific changes. Ask about all the key symptoms, including mood symptoms.

- *What happens when the medication wears off or is not taken?* Patients should be asked to compare days they have taken the medication with days the medication was omitted or forgotten. They can also be asked how they feel when the effects of the medication have worn off, for example in the evenings.

- *What side effects or unwanted effects are there?* Patients should be asked about specific important side effects, particulary those involving sleep, appetite, and mood.

Methylphenidate

Methylphenidate is a chain-substitute amphetamine derivative (Figure 7.2). It is available in the UK in two formulations: Immediate-release (IR) and ER. In the US, a transdermal patch has also been approved by the Food and Drug Administration (FDA), and this new formulation partially avoids first-pass metabolism, therefore resulting in a higher exposure to the drug.

Despite evidence proving the efficacy of methylphenidate in adults with ADHD [5,7,8,10], at the time of writing, in the UK and most of Europe, it is only licensed for first time use in for children and adolescents with ADHD. Recent meta-analyses found substantial effect sizes in the region of 0.5 or above (expressed as standard mean differences) [7,10,11].

Mechanism of action

Methylphenidate is a dopamine and noradrenaline reuptake inhibitor. It acts on both the prefrontal cortex and the subcortical striatum, modulating catecholaminergic tone. Its main action is through enhancement of dopamine signalling by blockade of the dopamine transporter, leading to increases in extracellular dopamine, as well as norepinephrine. It may also enhance the direct release of dopamine.

Methylphenidate may also have actions on other neurotransmitters, including histamine and serotonin.

Pharmacokinetics

Methylphenidate is easily absorbed orally, particularly if taken with food. It undergoes an important first-pass metabolism by de-esterification

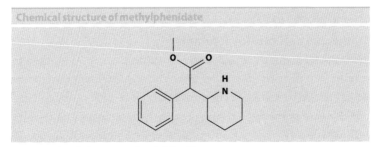

Chemical structure of methylphenidate

Figure 7.2 Chemical structure of methylphenidate.

in the gut, and only 30% of the oral dose is bioavailable. Peak plasma concentrations are reached 1 or 2 hours after oral administration, though this may vary according to whether it is an IR or ER preparation. Methylphenidate does not have any significant P450 interactions. It is eliminated by the kidneys as piperidine acetic acid, an inactive metabolite.

Side effects
The most frequently reported side effects are appetite loss, insomnia, headache, irritability, and tachycardia. Some side effects may disappear after 1 or 2 weeks of treatment (eg, headache, irritability), while insomnia and appetite loss may persist and may require dose reduction. Table 7.3 lists associated side effects (those with an asterisk affect more than 1 in 10 patients).

Contraindications and cautions
Susceptibility to angle-closure glaucoma is a caution in the use of methylphenidate. It should usually be avoided in patients with current drug or alcohol dependence; active psychosis; severe depression; anxiety or agitation; suicidal ideation; or anorexia nervosa. It is contraindicated in the presence of cardiovascular disease, including structural cardiac abnormalities, cerebrovascular disease, vasculitis, hyperthyroidism, or pheochromocytoma.

Methylphenidate may rarely produce tics or exacerbate existing tic disorders (such as Tourette's syndrome), and both the British National Formulary [12] and the FDA [13] advise caution in individuals with tic disorders. However, studies do not seem to support a worsening of tics in most children with ADHD and a comorbid tic disorder [14].

Stimulants and cardiovascular risk
Both methylphenidate and dexamphetamine are contraindicated in severe cardiovascular disease. NICE recommends that before treatment with stimulants is started, there is an evaluation of cardiovascular symptoms/disease in the individual (particularly hypertrophic obstructive cardiomyopathy), and a history taken of cardiovascular disease in family members (particularly a familial history of sudden death) [1].

Side effects associated with methylphenidate

Side effect	Comments
Cardiovascular	
Tachycardia and palpitations	Usually at the start of treatment, if the dosage is too high or if other stimulants (eg, caffeine, nicotine) are taken concurrently
Hypertension	Blood pressure usually only rises by about 5 mmHg. A key question is whether the patient already has hypertension or borderline hypertension
Angina	Rare
Myocardial infarction	Very rare
Neurological	
Insomnia*	Assess baseline sleep pattern. Many patients have insomnia before treatment is started and this may actually improve with treatment
	If there is initial insomnia, adjust regime so that medication is not given late in the day. However, some patients may sleep better if they take a small dose (eg, 5 mg) of instant-release in the evening
	If sleep is <5 hours per night, lower the dose
	Give sleep optimization advice; a low-dose tricyclic antidepressant may be useful; some use melatonin (however, this is not evidence-based)
Headache*	Patients with a history of migraine may be particularly vulnerable
	Use standard measures to manage headache
Tics	Very rare in adults without a history of Tourette's syndrome (and may be occuring due to undiagnosed Tourette's syndrome)
	Consider introducing medication to control tics or change to atomoxetine
Drowsiness	Due to the calming effect of the medication
Neuroleptic malignant syndrome	Very rare
Psychiatric	
Anxiety, nervousness, irritability, aggression* (continues overleaf)	Usually patients report feeling calmer on a stimulant
	Patients with comorbid somatic anxiety symptoms are particularly vulnerable to anxiety attacks when taking stimulants
	Determine whether this happens after taking medication or due to a return or exacerbation of the symptoms when the dose is wearing off (rebound symptoms)
	Use of methylphenidate may occasionally lead to feeling more irritable, angry or frustrated than usual

Table 7.3 Side effects associated with methylphenidate (continues overleaf).

Side effects associated with methylphenidate (continued)

Side effect	Comments
Psychiatric	
Anxiety, nervousness, irritability, aggression* (continued)	Patients may require more frequent dosing or change to an ER formulation, to avoid rebound symptoms in between doses of IR medication
	Effective strategies to limit adverse effects include reducing the dose at each dosing point, reduce dosing interval (if needed), or change to another medication
	Consider adding an antidepressant or anxiolytic (not a benzodiazepine) or try switching to atomoxetine
Depression	This needs to be differentiated from the mood instability of ADHD, as well as pre-existing comorbid depression
	Lower the dose of the stimulant
	Try a different stimulant or atomoxetine
	Consider adding in an antidepressant
	Consider cognitive behavioral therapy or other psychological interventions
Hypomania	Patients taking stimulants and antidepressants are at a higher risk
	Patients with a family history of bipolar disorder are at a higher risk
	Lower dose of medication or change to a nonstimulant
	If indicated, add a mood stabilizer
Psychosis	Rare, but patients with a past history of psychosis or borderline personality disorder are more vulnerable
	Stop the medication or, in very mild cases, consider a dose reduction
	Consider adding in an antipsychotic
Suicidal ideation	Very rare
Miscellaneous	Overmedicated patients may become withdrawn and under-responsive (a 'zombie'-like state). May also report being overly focused, unable to leave activities, or that they perseverate and become preoccupied with arranging and rearranging things. If this occurs, reduce the dose and review
Gastrointestinal	
Anorexia and weight loss	Get a baseline weight and monitor the weight throughout treatment
	Take medication with or after meals
	Increase size of meals when medication is not active (breakfast, dinner)
	Eat many small meals, finger foods and healthy snacks, and drink full-fat milk

Table 7.3 Side effects associated with methylphenidate (continues opposite).

Side effect	Comments
Gastrointestinal	
Abdominal pain	Stomach pains may improve after a snack or a drink (patients may be hungry without being aware of it)
	Take medication with or after meals
Nausea, dyspepsia	Often settles after the first 1 or 2 weeks of treatment or if medication is taken with food
Dry mouth	
Other uncommon side effects	
Urinary frequency	
Muscle cramps/tension	
Epistaxis	
Hematuria	
Blood disorders	
Excessive sweating	

Table 7.3 Side effects associated with methylphenidate (continued). Adapted from Concerta Prescribing Information [15].

Examination should include pulse rate and blood pressure (in addition to height, weight, and body mass index). Cardiovascular investigations (eg, electrocardiogram, echocardiogram) are only indicated where there is a personal or family history of cardiovascular disease or cardiovascular abnormalities on examination. Sudden death is no more common in patients taking stimulants than in the general population, except in patients with hypertrophic obstructive cardiomyopathy where the risk is significant [16]. Stimulants can be given to patients who have controlled hypertension. Table 7.4 provides a comparison of the effects of stimulants and nonstimulants on blood pressure, heart rate, and QTc interval and gives the relative rates of sudden death [16].

Medication	HR (bpm)	BP (mmHg)	QTc	Sudden death/ 100,000 patient years
Methylphenidate	↑ 6	↑ 5–10	None	0.2–0.5
Amphetamines	↑ 6	↑ 3–4	None	0.2–0.5
Atomoxetine	↑ 6	↑ 5–10	Caution	0.2–.0.5 perhaps 0

Table 7.4 Sudden deaths are no more common then the background population rate. BP, blood pressure; HR, heart rate. Reproduced with permission from Stiefel et al 2010 [16].

Stimulants and psychosis

Therapeutic doses of stimulants are occasionally implicated in causing psychosis with no previous history. In the US, the FDA rates this side effect as 'uncommon-rare.' High doses of amphetamines can produce psychotic symptoms indistinguishable from schizophrenia in predisposed patients. The risk of stimulant-induced psychosis in patients with a history of psychosis is greater. A systematic review showed 30% of patients with schizophrenia without active psychosis developed transient symptoms of an acute psychosis in response to stimulant use [17]. It is essential to screen for a past history of psychosis/psychotic illness and weigh up the risks and benefits of stimulant treatment.

Drug interactions

Methylphenidate should be used with caution in patients using monoamine oxidase inhibitors, dopaminergic drugs, and central alpha-adrenergic agonists. Methylphenidate inhibits the metabolism of tricyclic antidepressants [18], therefore downward dosage adjustment of these drugs may be required when given concomitantly with methylphenidate. Carbamazepine induces the metabolism of methylphenidate, decreasing its therapeutic effect.

Potential for abuse

Methylphenidate has been reported as a drug of abuse among US college students [19]. It theoretically has street value, though this is far more likely to be for its cognitive enhancement effects, rather that its ability to cause a 'high.' Methylphenidate does not cause tolerance or addiction when taken orally and within usual therapeutic doses. However, tolerance, addiction and psychological dependency may occur with regular use of high doses, especially if injected or snorted.

Methylphenidate is reported to be much less pleasurable than 'street' stimulants such as amphetamines and cocaine, which are known to produce a rapid feeling of euphoria [20]. This is partly due to the relatively slow absorption of an orally ingested tablet but also the fact that methylphenidate enters the brain more slowly than other drugs, causing a less sharp increase in dopamine [21]. The rate of entry of a substance in the brain determines its addictive potential. The faster the entry, the more addictive the drug is. This mechanism is key to the development of reinforcement and reward responses in addiction. The slow rate of entry of methylphenidate limits its potential for abuse [20].

One of the ER formulations of methylphenidate (Concerta XL) has an even lower abuse potential because the methylphenidate cannot be easily extracted for intravenous injection. IR formulations are not recommended in patients at risk of abuse but ER preparations can be considered. However, atomoxetine is normally considered first-line where drug abuse or diversion is considered a risk.

Summary of use

Methylphenidate is the first-line choice for the treatment of ADHD in adults in the UK. It is available in the UK as Ritalin®, Medikinet®, and Equasym®, (or generic preparations) in its short-acting form and Concerta® XL, Equasym XL®, and Medikinet retard® in its ER form. In the UK, methylphenidate (like the amphetamines) has been classified as a 'controlled drug,' and therefore prescriptions must be written in accordance with Department of Health guidance (outlined in the BNF) [12].

Methylphenidate is often initiated as an IR formulation, as this confers a greater degree of control during the titration period to establish the optimal dose. Once the patient is stable, they could be switched to an ER formulation if preferred. It should be noted, however, that ER preparations are significantly more expensive than IR ones. ER preparations are best selected as first choice where compliance with multiple dosing regimes is likely to be a problem. See Table 7.5 for comparison costs of ADHD medications [12]. Blood pressure, pulse, and weight need to be monitored when using this drug; this is usually done along with maintenance prescribing by the patient's general practitioner. Titration regimes (for guidance only) are shown in Table 7.6, and dosage equivalents of various preparations of methylphenidate (IR and ER) are shown in Table 7.7.

When using IR preparations, the typical starting dose for adults is 5 mg once- or twice-daily to allow the system to adjust to the medication gradually. This can be increased to 5 mg three times a day after

Costs for 28 days of attention deficit hyperactivity disorder medication		
Methylphenidate	Ritalin [nonproprietary]	30 mg/day=£17 100 mg/day=£48
Modified release methylphenidate	Concerta XL	27 mg/day=£37 108 mg/day=£127
	Equasym XL	30 mg/day=£35 100 mg/day=£130
	Medikinet retard XL	30 mg/day=£31 100 mg/day=£113
Dexamfetamine	[nonproprietary]	30 mg/day=£94
Atomoxetine	Strattera	80 mg/day=£83
Bupropion	Zyban	300 mg/day=£48
Modafinil	Provigil	400 mg/day=£210

Table 7.5 Costs for 28 days of attention deficit hyperactivity disorder medication. Adapted from BNF [12].

approximately a week. Thereafter, the dosage can be increased as required and tolerated by about 10–15 mg daily per week to a maximum of 100 mg daily. When using ER preparations, start at 10 mg (or 18 mg, if using Concerta XL) once-daily, increasing to 20 mg (27 or 36 mg, if Concerta XL) after 1 week, increasing by 10–20 mg (or 18 mg if Concerta XL) daily about every 1 to 2 weeks as required and tolerated, up to a maximum of 100 mg (or 108 mg, if Concerta XL - see guidance in Table 7.4). It is sensible to titrate more slowly and review between no more than two stepwise increases to avoid any unnecessary side effects. Follow up should be weekly, fortnightly, or monthly as required and, with experience, may be via telephone at times. The treatment should be discontinued if there is no response after a month, with titration to higher doses. In order to assess the condition, the medication should be stopped for a few weeks every 1 or 2 years.

The duration of action of IR preparations varies between individuals but is usually in the region of 3 or 4 hours, allowing dosing at breakfast (eg, 9 am), lunch (eg, 1 pm), and tea time (eg, 5 pm). A fourth dose (taken in the evening) can be given, particularly if the individual needs to be symptom-free at this time of day. To avoid any potential risk of tolerance, it is best to have a 12-hour nighttime 'wash out' period during which the drug is not active. In addition, taking the medication too close to a patient's bedtime may result in sleep difficulties in some individuals.

Titration regimes for methylphenidate

Formulation	Regime	Morning dose (eg, 9am, taken with breakfast)	Lunch-time dose (eg, 1pm, taken with lunch)	Tea-time dose (eg, 5pm, ideally taken with a snack)
IR	Low	5 mg	5 mg	5 mg
	Average	10 mg	10 mg	10 mg
	Average	15 mg	15 mg	15 mg
	Average-high	20 mg	20 mg	20 mg
	High	25 mg	25 mg	25 mg
	High	30 mg	30 mg	30 mg
ER (Concerta XL)	Low	18 mg		+/– IR (eg, 5 mg)
	Low	27 mg		+/– IR
	Average	36 mg		+/– IR
	Average	54 mg*		+/– IR
	Average-High	72 mg*		+/– IR
	High	90 mg*,†		+/– IR

Table 7.6 **Titration regimes for methylphenidate.** IR, instant-release; ER, extended-release. *These doses need to be made up of combinations of the above tablets; †The maximum dose of Concerta XL in randomized controlled trials is 72 mg but many clinicians go as high as 108 mg. This practice is not formally recommended by the manufacturer but is commonly practiced.

Dosage equivalents of the instant-release formulation of methylphenidate and three brands of extended-release methylphenidate

IR formulation (total daily dose)	Concerta XL	Equasym XL	Medikinet Retard
10 mg	—	10 mg	10 mg
15 mg	18 mg	—	—
20 mg	27 mg	20 mg	20 mg
30 mg	36 mg	30 mg	30 mg
40 mg	—	—	40 mg
45 mg	54 mg	—	—
60 mg	72 mg	60 mg	—

Table 7.7 **Dosage equivalents of the instant-release formulation of methylphenidate and three brands of extended-release methylphenidate.**

In others, however, a small dose (eg, 5 mg) taken before bedtime has the paradoxical effect of improving sleep due to better control of symptoms and has not been reported to lead to tolerance.

The duration of action of ER preparation varies, as does the pattern of release. In all three cases, a percentage of the dose is released immediately following ingestion, with the rest being gradually released thereafter.

See Table 7.8 to compare the pattern of release and duration of action of the three ER preparations. ER preparations (eg, Medikinet, Equasym, Concerta) sometimes need to be taken twice daily where symptom control is required throughout the day and evening.

Amphetamines

Amphetamines belong to the phenethylamine family (Figure 7.3). Four different amphetamines have been used in ADHD: levamphetamine (levoamphetamine), dexamphetamine (dextroamphetamine), methamphetamine, and lisdexamphetamine.

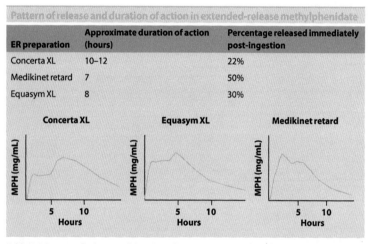

Pattern of release and duration of action in extended-release methylphenidate

ER preparation	Approximate duration of action (hours)	Percentage released immediately post-ingestion
Concerta XL	10–12	22%
Medikinet retard	7	50%
Equasym XL	8	30%

Table 7.8 **Pattern of release and duration of action in extended-release methylphenidate.** Adapted from Banaschewski et al [22].

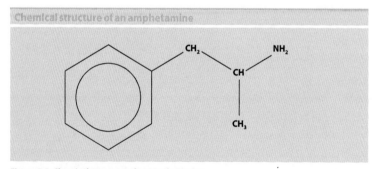

Figure 7.3 **Chemical structure of an amphetamine.**

Adderall® (mixed amphetamine salts) is a preparation widely used in the US but not available in the UK. The ER pro-drug lisdexamphetamine (Vyvanse) is a useful alternative, although at the time or writing, is not yet licensed in Europe. In the UK and some other parts of Europe, generic dexamphetamine is available as an alternative IR medication to methylphenidate. Dexamphetamine has shown efficacy in one randomized placebo-controlled trial in adults with ADHD [23] and an open study lasting more than 31 weeks [24]. More evidence is available for mixed amphetamine salts, which show efficacy that is similar to that of other stimulants [5].

Mechanism of action

Amphetamines have a dual action in the neuron, both of which increase synaptic noradrenaline and dopamine availability:

- blockade of reuptake of dopamine and noradrenaline by competitive inhibition of the transporters (dopamine active transporter [DAT] and norepinephrine transporter [NAT]);
- promotion of release of dopamine and noradrenaline by competitive inhibition of the intraneuronal vesicular monoamine transporter (VMAT).

The second of these actions is particularly relevant when amphetamines are used as a drug of abuse [24]. At high doses, amphetamines have a serotonergic effect.

Pharmacokinetics

Dexamphetamine is easily absorbed by the small intestine and rapidly distributed to body tissues. About 30% is eliminated unchanged by the renal system, the remainder being metabolized in the liver, primarily by the P450 2D6 enzyme system.

Lisdexamphetamine has similar pharmacokinetics to those of dexamphetamine, with one major difference: lisdexamphetamine is a prodrug (ie, it is inactive). After absorption by the small intestine, the L-lysine portion of the molecule is cleaved off, leaving the active substance dexamphetamine. The conversion is facilitated by enzymes in the heme element of red blood cells [25]. Lisdexamphetamine has a longer duration of action, and it is less easily abusable. The beneficial effects of amphetamines commence within an hour of ingestion and peak after 2 or 3 hours, with a total duration of action of 4–7 hours [25].

Side effects

Possible side effects of amphetamines are summarized in Table 7.9. The side-effect profile of amphetamines is similar to that of methylphenidate (Table 7.3), with the most commonly reported side effects being insomnia and restlessness.

Contraindications and cautions

Contraindications include cardiovascular disease (eg, moderate-to-severe hypertension, cardiomyopathy, arrhythmia, family history of sudden death), hyperexcitability or agitated states, hyperthyroidism, and glaucoma. Like methylphenidate, amphetamines are usually avoided when

Side effects of amphetamines	
Cardiovascular	Tachycardia, palpitations
	Angina
	Increased blood pressure
	Cardiomyopathy
Neurological/psychiatric	Insomnia
	Restlessness
	Irritability
	Excitability
	Nervousness
	Euphoria
	Convulsions
	Tremor
	Choreoathetoid movements
	Dizziness
	Headache
	Tics and Tourette's symptoms (in predisposed patients)
	Psychosis
Gastrointestinal	Anorexia and weight loss
	Dry mouth
Other	Sweating
	Glaucoma

Table 7.9 Side effects of amphetamines.

there is potential for abuse or diversion. See Chapter 10 for guidance on prescribing in pregnancy. The risks and benefits of treatment must be weighed up in patients with a past history of psychosis (see section on stimulants and psychosis on page 98).

Amphetamines have been linked to reports of sudden death in children [26]. This led to the temporary suspension of the license for mixed amphetamine salts in Canada in 2004. Two 2011 epidemiological studies of adults/teenagers with ADHD taking stimulant medication failed to show any increase in sudden death, stroke, or myocardial infarction in this population [27,28]. The FDA has maintained a general recommendation of monitoring pulse and blood pressure in all patients treated with stimulant medication, but no further monitoring tests are required [13].

Drug interactions

A number of coprescribed drugs can interact with amphetamines (Table 7.10). Alkalinization or acidification of the urine can moderate the efficiency of renal excretion of amphetamines (which accounts for 30% of their elimination) agents that acidify the urine tend to increase the rate of renal excretion.

As mentioned above, amphetamine compounds are substrates of the enzyme system CYP2D6. Drugs that inhibit this system (eg, fluoxetine, paroxetine, tricyclic antidepressants, cocaine) may increase plasma levels of dexamphetamine. Drugs that induce the CYP2D6 system (eg, carbamazepine) will decrease plasma levels of dexamphetamine. As amphetamines have several potential metabolic pathways available to them, the impact of inhibition or induction of CYP2D6 by coprescribed drugs is less than with drugs that have only a single metabolic route. Thus, CYP2D6 inhibitors and inducers usually have only a moderate effect on the bioavailability of the drug, unless other relevant CYP enzymes are simultaneously affected.

Potential for abuse

Amphetamines are associated with tolerance and addiction, when taken in high doses (particularly when snorted or injected), which is typical of many abused substances. Consequently, they are not recommended as a first-line

Summary of interactions of amphetamines	
Selective serotonin re-uptake inhibitors (SSRIs)	Possible increase in plasma levels of amphetamines and hypertensive crisis
Tricyclic antidepressants (TCAs)	Possible increase in plasma levels of amphetamines and hypertensive crisis
Monoamine oxidase inhibitors (MAO) inhibitors	Possible increase in plasma levels of amphetamines and hypertensive crisis
Carbamazepine	Possible decrease in plasma levels of amphetamines
Typical antipsychotics (haloperidol+phenothiazines – eg, chlorpromazine trifluoperazine)	Due to reduction in dopamine levels, may diminish effect of amphetamines
Propranolol	As propanolol works by blocking adrenaline, its effects may be diminished when using amphetamines causing hypertension
Dopaminergic agents	Additive effect – potential caution
Noradrenergic agents	Additive effect – potential caution
Gastric acidifying agents (eg, ascorbic acid)	Decreased absorption of amphetamines
Gastric alkalizing agents (eg, acetazolamide)	Increased absorption of amphetamines
Urinary acidifying agents (eg, ascorbic acid)	Increased excretion of amphetamines
Urinary alkalizing agents (eg, sodium citrate)	Decreased excretion of amphetamines

Table 7.10 Summary of interactions of amphetamines.

treatment in patients where abuse or diversion are considered potential risks. Aside from diversion for cognitive enhancement, the key concern is that tablets will be crushed and then snorted or injected, increasing the speed of entry of the drug into the brain, and achieving a 'high.' For these reasons, amphetamines have a street value. Thus, dosage and dispensation of the drug should be carefully monitored, and prescriptions should be stopped if there is a suspicion of misuse.

Lisdexamphetamine is a good alternative associated with a negligible risk of abuse even when injected, owing to its pharmacokinetic properties – when it is injected intravenously, the active compound is released slowly from the inactive component – meaning there is no rapid peak in plasma concentration and brain entry. Consequently, it does not produce the fast euphoric reaction associated with IR dexamphetamine.

Summary of use

In the US, amphetamines are available in four formulations:

- methamphetamine (Dexosyn®);
- mixed amphetamine salts containing, amongst other things, levamphetamine and dexamphetamine (Adderall®);
- dexamphetamine (Dexedrine®);
- lisdexamphetamine (Vyvanse®).

At the time of writing, in the UK and most of Europe, only generic dexamphetamine is licensed; however Vyvanse can be imported at comparable cost to other extended release drugs for ADHD, and is starting to be used (off-label) in the UK. Under British Law, amphetamines, like methylphenidate, have been classified as 'controlled drugs' regardless of formulation, and therefore prescriptions must be written in accordance with Department of Health guidance (outlined in the BNF) [12].

Titration regimes (for guidance only) are shown in Table 7.11. Dexamphetamine should be started at 5 mg once-daily and uptitrated according to response and tolerability following similar procedures to methylphenidate. Once titrated up, it is usually given two or three times a day, up to a maximum daily dose of 60 mg. Dexamphetamine IR has a slightly longer duration of action that Methylphenidate IR.

In summary, amphetamines are an effective treatment for ADHD in adults. Abuse potential is similar or slightly higher than methylphenidate, although the pro-drug lisdexamphetamine has a neglible risk for tolerance or addiction. As is the case for methylphenidate, cardiovascular illness and any previous history of psychosis needs to be assessed and the risks and benefits weighed up carefully before treatment is started. To date, amphetamines are not regarded as first-line treatment in the UK, where

Typical titration regimes for dexamphetamine

Regime	Morning dose (mg)	Lunch-time dose (mg)	Tea-time dose (mg)
Low	5 mg	5 mg	—
Low	5 mg	5 mg	5 mg
Average	10 mg	10 mg	10 mg
Average–high	15 mg	15 mg	15 mg
High	20 mg	20 mg	20 mg

Table 7.11 Typical titration regimes for dexamphetamine.

methylphenidate is preferred [1]. However, their efficacy is thought to be similar to methylphenidate and slightly greater than the equivalent nonstimulant alternatives.

Table 7.12 is a summary checklist that can be used before initiating treatment with any stimulant medication.

Atomoxetine

The nonstimulant atomoxetine is well-established as a second-line drug treatment for ADHD in both children and adults. Unlike stimulants, atomoxetine is not a controlled medication. The drug acts as a specific noradrenergic reuptake inhibitor (NARI) and has some similarities to antidepressants with a delayed onset of action. Despite this, previous studies have found that atomoxetine has no antidepressant effects. It is generally given as a once-daily dose (but can be given twice-daily to improve efficacy or tolerability) and comes in the form of hard capsules that can be taken with or without food.

Randomized controlled trials in adults support the use of atomoxetine in ADHD [29–31], with effect sizes averaging around 0.4 (Cohen d) and a number needed to treat (NNT) of around 5. Two trials comparing atomoxetine with methylphenidate in children showed similar efficacy to methylphenidate IR preparations, but a smaller effect size than methylphenidate ER [32–34]. Overall, the superiority of methylphenidate to atomoxetine in terms of effect size is not well-established. However, in

Checklist for the initiation of stimulant medication	
Personal medical history	Psychotic illness
	Medication and/or substance abuse
	Cardiovascular disease
	General medical health, particularly with regard to other medications that will be taken simultaneously, especially those with cardiovascular effects
Family history	Cardiovascular disease, particularly early onset or a history of sudden death
General examination	Obtain baseline weight, height, and body mass index
Cardiovascular examination	A basic cardiovascular examination including auscultation, pulse rate, and blood pressure

Table 7.12 Checklist for the initiation of stimulant medication. Adapted from NICE [1].

all trials the dropout rate due to side effects is greater with atomoxetine than stimulants.

Mechanism of action

Atomoxetine is a highly selective noradrenaline reuptake inhibitor. It blocks the presynaptic noradrenaline transporter and has two main effects in the brain:

- increases the availability of noradrenaline in the synapse;
- increases synaptic dopamine in the prefrontal cortex
  (as dopamine is normally taken up by the noradrenaline
  transporter in this region).

Pharmacokinetics

Atomoxetine is well absorbed from the digestive tract after oral administration, reaching peak plasma concentrations 1 or 2 hours after dosing [35]. It is almost completely bound to plasma proteins, primarily albumin. It is metabolized in the liver (with only modest first-pass metabolism) and the metabolites are excreted renally in the urine.

Atomoxetine is mainly metabolized by the CYP2D6 enzymatic pathway. About 7% of the Caucasian population and 2% of the Asian population have mutations or deletions in genes that codify this cytochrome and are considered 'poor metabolizers,' having a several-fold higher exposure to plasma concentration of atomoxetine [36]. In normal 'extensive' metabolizers, atomoxetine-derived compounds are completely eliminated 24 hours after the last dose. In poor metabolizers, however, this process may take 72 hours or more. The higher concentrations of atomoxetine in the plasma and longer duration of action, lead to more side effects and greater risk of harm in the case of overdose.

Side effects

Common side effects with atomoxetine include gastrointestinal symptoms (eg, nausea, vomiting, reduced appetite, abdominal pain, and constipation), insomnia, dry mouth, dizziness, and headache. Reduced libido and other sexual side effects are commonly reported [35]. Some people report tachycardia, palpitations, hot flushes, and urinary symptoms. Many of these unwanted effects will disappear in the first weeks of treatment and can often be avoided by gradual up-titration of dose.

Many patients experience a modest increase in pulse (mean <10 beats/minute) and/or increase in blood pressure (mean <5 mmHg), which for most people is not clinically significant. Caution is advised where there is pre-existing hypertension, tachycardia, cardiovascular, or cerebrovascular disease. Regardless, pulse and blood pressure should be measured periodically, particularly after dose changes whilst taking the medication.

Increased incidence of suicidal thoughts has been reported with this drug but is uncommon. Patients need to be informed of this risk, and suicidal ideation should be monitored for, especially in the early phase of treatment.

There have been rare case reports of acute liver disease following administration of atomoxetine [35]. Patients should be informed of the cardinal symptoms of liver failure (abdominal pain, jaundice, unexplained nausea) and these features or elevated hepatic enzymes or bilirubin should prompt immediate medical review and discontinuation of the medication. Both seizures and treatment-emergent psychotic or manic symptoms can also result from treatment with atomoxetine and caution is advised.

The NICE guidelines recommend monitoring of weight, heart rate, and blood pressure before and after every dose change [1]. Weight should be measured every 6 months once the patient is on a stable dose; however, weight changes are not usually a long-term problem. Heart rate and blood pressure should ideally be recorded every 3 months. The side effects of atomoxetine are summarized in Table 7.13.

Contraindications and cautions

Atomoxetine is contraindicated in narrow-angle glaucoma. It also should not be used in combination with, or within 2 weeks of, monoamine oxidase inhibitors.

Drug interactions

As mentioned above, atomoxetine should not be used with monoamine oxidase inhibitors. Additionally, atomoxetine is primarily metabolized by the CYP2D6 pathway and potent inhibitors of CYP2D6 increase atomoxetine concentrations in plasma similar to those observed in CYP2D6 poor metabolizer patients. Paroxetine is a strong inhibitor of CYP2D6, and fluoxetine, is a relatively strong inhibitor of the cytochrome.

Side effects of atomoxetine	
Gastrointestinal	Liver disease (rare)
	Reduced appetite*
	Dry mouth*
	Nausea and vomiting*
	Constipation
	Abdominal pain
	Dyspepsia
Neurological/psychiatric	Suicidal ideation (rare)
	Sleep disturbance*
	Dizziness
	Headache
	Lethargy/fatigue
	Mood swings*
	Anxiety*
	Irritability/aggression*
	Seizures
Ophthalmological	Glaucoma (contraindication)
	Mydriasis
Dermatological	Rash
	Dermatitis
	Pruritus
	Excessive sweating
Cardiovascular	Hot flushes
	Palpitations
	Tachycardia
	Increased blood pressure
	Postural hypotension*
Other	Urinary hesitancy / retention
	Dysuria
	Prostatitis
	Sexual dysfunction
	Menstrual disturbances

Table 7.13 **Side effects of atomoxetine.** *Very common, affect more than 1 in 10 patients. Adapted from Strattera SPC [35].

Atomoxetine itself does not cause significant inhibition or induction of cytochrome P450 enzymes.

The drugs listed in Table 7.14 are CYP2D6 substrates that can act as competitive inhibitors. For an exhaustive list of inhibitors and inducers of liver cytochromes, see Bazire 2011 [18].

Despite potential for antagonism, it is possible to use treatments for ADHD and antipsychotics effectively at the same time. Drugs that affect noradrenaline (eg, antidepressants such as imipramine, venlafaxine, mirtazapine, or decongestants such as pseudoephedrine and phenylephrine) should be used cautiously with atomoxetine due to the additive effect.

An increased risk of ventricular arrhythmias has been described when using atomoxetine with drugs that prolong the QT interval (eg, antipsychotics, methadone, tricyclic antidepressants, lithium) [18]. Drugs that lower the seizure threshold (eg, some antipsychotics, buproprion, tricyclic antidepressants) may increase the risk of seizures when given together with atomoxetine.

Use caution when using salbutamol (high-dose nebulized or systemically administered intravenously or orally) together with atomoxetine, as the effect of salbutamol on the cardiovascular system can be potentiated.

Inhibitors of the CYP2D6 complex	
Strong inhibitors	Fluoxetine
	Norfluoxetine
	Paroxetine
Moderate and weak inhibitors	Bupropion
	Modafinil
	Duloxetine
	Escitalopram
	Haloperidol
	Chlorpromazine
	Clomipramine
	Amiodarone
	Chloroquine
	Cimetidine
	Cocaine

Table 7.14 Inhibitors of the CYP2D6 complex. Adapted from Bazire et al [18].

Potential for abuse

Atomoxetine has extremely low abuse potential and is not associated with euphoriant properties and therefore it is generally considered the first-line treatment in patients with substance misuse problems.

Summary of use

Atomoxetine is not a controlled drug in the UK. Because of its low abuse potential, it a good option for patients with a history of substance abuse. Otherwise, it is considered a second-line treatment for use when no improvement has been observed with an adequate trial of methylphenidate (6 weeks) or when the patient has developed side effects that prevent further treatment with stimulants.

In general, it is initiated by clinicians experienced in the treatment of ADHD but can be continued by a general practitioner, with an annual review by the specialist, once the patient is on a stable dose. Unlike stimulants the initiation typically follows a standard protocol and does not require the same degree of individualized 'fine tuning' of the dose.

Dosing

In patients with a body weight over 70 kg, the initial total daily dosage is 40 mg for a minimum of 1 week, before being cautiously increased according to response and tolerability to a maximum of 100 mg daily. The usual maintenance dose is 80 mg daily and no additional benefit has been demonstrated for doses higher than this. Increasing the dose by 20 mg each week from 40 mg is a sensible and cautious approach, potentially minimizing side effects. Even much more cautious dose titration (and lower maintenance doses) should be used in those suspected of being 'poor metabolizers.' In patients with a body weight under 70 kg, atomoxetine should be initiated at a total daily dose of 0.5 mg/kg, again increasing cautiously and gradually after at least 7 days to a maintenance dose of approximately 1.2 mg/kg. Heart rate, blood pressure, and weight should be monitored before and during treatment (especially at every dose change). Patients should be warned about the potential suicidal thoughts and liver complications, even though they are rare.

Bupropion

Bupropion is a noradrenaline and dopamine reuptake inhibitor and it is considered to be a mild psychostimulant due to its amphetamine-derived chemical structure. It is only approved in the UK for use as a smoking cessation agent (eg, Zyban®). In the US, it is also licensed for the treatment of ADHD and depression (eg, Wellbutrin®, Zyban®, Voxra®, Budeprion®, or Aplenzin®). Bupropion is sometimes used (off-label) as a third-line drug in ADHD when stimulants and atomoxetine have failed to improve symptoms or they have not been tolerated. It is a useful consideration when the ADHD is relatively mild with less profound effects or if the patient is also keen to give up smoking.

A number of RCTs [37] have reported benefit with bupropion for ADHD, although effects were less pronounced than with methylphenidate. In a recent meta-analysis, patients taking bupropion were 2.4 times more likely to report improvement than patients on placebo [37]. However, this result should be interpreted with caution as the studies pooled were very heterogeneous and had small sample sizes.

Pharmacokinetics

Bupropion is rapidly absorbed by the digestive system and its concentration peaks in the plasma within 2 hours of oral ingestion. It has a half-life of 14 hours. ER formulations prolong the half-life further.

Side effects

Rarely, serious side effects can occur, including seizures (bupropion reduces the seizure threshold and caution is required when using other drugs that do this), anaphylaxis, psychosis, mania, and suicidal ideation. Cardiovascular side effects can also occur.

Contraindications

Bupropion is contraindicated in patients with a previous history of bipolar disorder, an eating disorder, or seizures (or conditions that reduce the seizure threshold such as alcohol or benzodiazepine withdrawal). It should be used with caution in liver or renal impairment and severe hypertension. It also should not be used in combination with, or within 2 weeks of using, monoamine oxidase inhibitors.

Drug interactions

Bupropion is metabolized by the CYP2B6 enzyme and therefore CYP2B6 inhibitors (eg, paroxetine, fluoxetine, fluvoxamine, and clopidogrel) may increase its plasma levels. CYP2B6 inducers (eg, efavirenz, modafinil, and rifampicin) have the reverse effect. Bupropion is itself a moderately strong inhibitor of CYP2D6, which metabolizes atomoxetine and venlafaxine (and to a lesser extent, amphetamine). Combinations of these drugs are not recommended as they can potentially increase side effects. As it is a dopaminergic agent, bupropion should be used with caution with levodopa and other substances that increase dopamine availability.

As bupropion lowers the seizure threshold, it should not be used with other medications that also lower the seizure threshold. Caution should be exercised when using bupropion with alcohol, as it may reduce alcohol tolerance.

Potential for abuse

Anecdotal reports of bupropion as a recreational drug exist [38], but it is not a controlled drug and can be prescribed to patients with a history of drug abuse.

Summary of use

Randomized control trials of bupropion in ADHD have used daily doses varying between 200 mg and 400 mg [37]. In the UK, the most commonly available bupropion preparation is Zyban (150 mg ER tablets). If using this, it is recommended to start at 150 mg once-daily, and wait at least 1 week before considering an increase to 150 mg twice-daily [12]. Careful monitoring of side effects, particularly raised blood pressure, is required. If seizures occur, the drug should be discontinued.

Bupropion has been proved to be beneficial in adults with ADHD [37], but evidence is still limited and it probably should not be used as a first-line medication. It can be a useful option when other medications (eg, methylphenidate, dexamphetamine, atomoxetine) have not succeeded in controlling symptoms or are not tolerated.

Other substances

Modafinil

Modafinil is a 'wakefulness-promoting substance' used in narcolepsy. Its precise mechanism of action is unknown but it appears to increase the production of histamine and orexin by stimulating the hypothalamus and may also increase dopamine and noradrenaline. Modafinil is not a controlled drug in the UK. Use in ADHD is exclusively off-label.

In a recent review of the efficacy of modafinil versus placebo in ADHD, the reduction of ADHD symptoms was summarized as being clinically meaningful but statistically modest and far less than that accomplished with classic stimulants [39].

Modafinil may reduce the effectiveness of oral contraceptives. Potential serious adverse reactions include severe rashes, Stevens-Johnson syndrome, and toxic epidermal necrolysis. It remains difficult to predict the severity of a rash when it starts, so patients need to be advised to discontinue modafinil if a rash occurs. Psychiatric side effects can include anxiety, irritability, hallucinations, and psychoses. Other side effects include gastrointestinal disturbance, tachycardia, sleep disruption, drowsiness, and visual symptoms.

Modafinil should not be used in moderate-to-severe hypertension or in severe cardiovascular disease. Addictive potential has been described in animals [40], and therefore caution should be used if prescribed to patients with a past history of drug abuse.

In summary, modafinil can be used with caution as a third-line agent in patients who have not responded to any other stimulant or atomoxetine, but prescribers should be specialists (or guided by specialists) in adult ADHD.

Alpha-2 adrenergic agonists

Clonidine and guanfacine are alpha-2 adrenergic agonists that are approved for the treatment of hypertension, although they are now rarely used for this indication due to their side effects, which include light headedness, dry mouth, dizziness, and constipation. In 2010, the FDA approved the use of clonidine as a monotherapy or as an adjunct to traditional stimulant treatment for ADHD. It can be particularly useful in patients with comorbid Tourette's syndrome.

The FDA has also approved an ER formulation of guanfacine (Intuniv®) for children and adolescents. Neither clonidine nor guanfacine are approved in the UK for this use but may have a place in patients with ADHD who have hypertension and therefore may have problems with stimulants and atomoxetine. Treatment with these medications should be guided by ADHD specialists.

Tricyclic antidepressants

Efficacy in ADHD has been described both with desipramine and nortryptiline, albeit mostly in combination with stimulant medications [41]. These substances may be useful to control some specific symptoms, for instance ADHD-like stimulant-induced insomnia and weight loss. Tricyclic antidepressants have very limited addictive potential. However, the cardiovascular risk associated with tricyclic antidepressants and their toxicity in overdose limit their use in patients with ADHD.

Selective serotonin reuptake inhibitors and serotonin and noradrenaline reuptake inhibitors

Selective serotonin reuptake inhibitors have not been found beneficial in the management of ADHD in the absence of any depressive symptoms.

One small RCT in adults and several in children have reported positive effects of venlafaxine in ADHD [42,43]. However, further research is necessary to estimate the real effect size of treatment with serotonin/noradrenaline reuptake inhibitors in the absence of depression. There is currently no trial evidence for other licensed serotonin/noradrenaline reuptake inhibitors such as duloxetine.

Antipsychotics

NICE guidelines do not recommend the routine use of antipsychotics for the treatment of ADHD [1]. However, low doses may be useful to control impulsivity and agitation in selected cases for limited periods of time, and may be considered in treatment-resistant cases.

Combination treatment

There is little evidence of the efficacy of combining drugs (or for combining different formulations of the same drug) for the treatment of ADHD in adults. In clinical practice, combination of IR and ER formulations of methylphenidate is common. The objective of this prescribing pattern is to maintain a continuous base level of methylphenidate in the blood by 'topping up' with an IR formulation when the ER concentration is decreasing, hence avoiding adding a dose of an ER preparation that may affect sleep.

Combinations of methylphenidate and atomoxetine are also occasionally seen in clinical practice [44]. This combination can be useful when the patient has been found to benefit from stimulant treatment but has difficulty tolerating it. Adding atomoxetine may allow a reduction in the dose of methylphenidate. However, no trials have been performed using this combination in adults with ADHD and it should probably be reserved for specialist clinics.

Prescription of methylphenidate in conjunction with amphetamine is not recommended, since both have cardiovascular risks and a similar side effect profile.

So, in summary, should stimulant treatment not be successful, prescribing atomoxetine is usually the next step. Should monotherapy with stimulants or atomoxetine prove to be ineffective or is not tolerated, one of the third-line drugs can be considered. An alternative could be a combination of ER and IR stimulants or a combination of stimulants and atomoxetine.

Before starting such a combination, it is important to have ensured that sufficient doses of the individual drugs have been taken for a sufficient period of time. A combination treatment may be beneficial for patients who do not tolerate high doses of one of the drugs because of side effects. However, there is a lack of trial data regarding such combinations and, in general, they should be reserved for those with specialist expertise in the condition.

It is also important to question the accuracy of the diagnosis, to explore whether there is active substance misuse and to consider non-pharmacological strategies (eg, psychotherapy, coaching) in patients who do not respond sufficiently to drug treatment (see Chapter 8).

References

1   National Institute for Health and Clinical Excellence (NICE). Attention Deficit Hyperactivity Disorder: NICE Guideline on Diagnosis and Management of ADHD in Children, Young People and Adults. NICE website. www.nice.org.uk/nicemedia/pdf/CG72NiceGuidelinev3.pdf. Accessed August 25, 2012.

2   Nutt DJ, Fone K, Asherson P, et al. Evidence-based guidelines for management of attention-deficit/hyperactivity disorder in adolescents in transition to adult services and in adults: recommendations from the British Association for Psychopharmacology. J Psychopharmacol. 2007;21:10-41.

3   Kooij S. Adult ADHD Diagnostic Assessment and Treatment. Amsterdam: Pearson; 2010.

4   Kooij SJ, Bejerot S, Blackwell A, et al. European consensus statement on diagnosis and treatment of adult ADHD: The European Network Adult ADHD. BMC Psychiatry. 2010;10:67.

5   Mészáros A, Czobor P, Bálint S, Komlósi S, Simon V, Bitter I. Pharmacotherapy of adult attention deficit hyperactivity disorder (ADHD): a meta-analysis. Int J Neuropsychopharmacol. 2009;12:1137-1147.

6   Wilens TE, Adler LA, Weiss MD, et al. Atomoxetine treatment of adults with ADHD and comorbid alcohol use disorders. Drug Alcohol Depend. 2008;96:145-154.

7   Koesters M, Becker T, Kilian R, Fergert JM, Weinmann S. Limits of meta-analysis: methylphenidate in the treatment of adult attention-deficit hyperactivity disorder. J Psychopharmacol. 2009;23:733-744.

8   Farone SV, Spencer T, Aleardi M, Pagano C, Biederman J. Meta-analysis of the efficacy of methylphenidate for treating adult attention-deficit/hyperactivity disorder. J Clin Psychopharmacol. 2004;24:24-29.

9   Michelson D, Adler L, Spencer T, et al. Atomoxetine in adults with ADHD: two randomized, placebo-controlled studies. Biol Psychiatry. 2003;53:112-120.

10 Castells X, Ramos-Quiroga JA, Rigau D, et al. Efficacy of methylphenidate for adults with attention-deficit hyperactivity disorder: a meta-regression analysis. CNS Drugs. 2011;25:157-169.

11 Faraone SV, Glatt SJ. A comparison of the efficacy of medications for adult attention-deficit/hyperactivity disorder using meta-analysis of effect sizes. J Clin Psychiatry. 2010;71:754-763.

12 British National Formulary (BNF). Methylphenidate hydrochloride. BNF website. www.bnf.org/bnf/bnf/current/86032.htm?q=methylphenidate&t=search&ss=text&p=3#_86032. Accessed August 25, 2012.

13 Food and Drug Administration (FDA). FDA Drug Safety Communication: Safety Review Update of Medications used to treat Attention-Deficit/Hyperactivity Disorder (ADHD) in adults. FDA website. www.fda.gov/Drugs/DrugSafety/ucm279858.htm. Accessed August 25, 2012.

14 Poncin Y, Sukhodolsky DG, McGuire J, Scahill L. Drug and non-drug treatments of children with ADHD and tic disorders. Eur Child Adolesc Psychiatry. 2007;16(suppl 1):78-88.

15 Concerta Extended Release Prescribing Information. Titusville, NJ: McNeil Pediatrics. www.concerta.net/sites/default/files/pdf/Prescribing_Info-short.pdf#zoom=56. Accessed August 25, 2012.

16 Stifel G, Besag FM. Cardiovascular effects of methylphenidate, amphetamines and atomoxetine in the treatment of attention-deficit hyperactivity disorder. Drug Saf. 2010;33:821-842.

17 Curran C, Byrappa N, McBride A. Stimulant psychosis: systematic review. Br J Psychiatry. 2004;185:196-204.

18 Bazire S. Psychotropic Drug Directory 2010: the Professionals' Pocket Handbook and Aide Memoire. Aberdeen: HealthComm UK; 2011.

19 McCabe SE, Knight JR, Teter CJ, Wechsler H. Non-medical use of prescription stimulants among US college students: prevalence and correlates from a national survey. Addiction. 2005;100:96-106.

20 Volkow ND, Ding YS, Fowler JS, et al. Is methylphenidate like cocaine? Studies on their pharmacokinetics and distribution in the human brain. Arch Gen Psychiatry. 1995;52:456-463.

21 Weikop P, Egestad B, Kehr J. Application of triple-probe microdialysis for fast pharmacokinetic/pharmacodynamic evaluation of dopamimetic activity of drug candidates in the rat brain. *J Neurosci Methods*. 2004;140:59-65.

22 Banaschewski T, Coghill D, Santosh P, et al. Long acting medications for the hyperkinetic disorders: a systematic review and European treatment guidelines. *Eur Child Adolesc Psychiatry*. 2006;15:476-495.

23 Spencer TJ, Adler LA, Weisler RH, Youcha SH. Triple-bead mixed amphetamine salts (SPD465), a novel, enhanced ER amphetamine formulation for the treatment of adults with ADHD: a randomized, double-blind, multicenter, placebo-controlled study. *J Clin Psychiatry*. 2008;69:1437-1448.

24 Stahl SM, Mignon L. *Stahl's Illustrated Attention Deficit Hyperactivity Disorder*. New York: Cambridge University Press; 2009.

25 Pennick M. Absorption of lisdexamphetamine dimesylate and its enzymatic conversion to d-amphetamine. *Neuropsychiatr Dis Treat*. 2010;6:317-327.

26 Silva RR, Skimming JW, Muniz R. Cardiovascular safety of stimulant medications for pediatric attention-deficit hyperactivity disorder. *Clin Pediatr (Phila)*. 2010;49:840-851.

27 Cooper WO, Habel LA, Sox CM, et al. ADHD drugs and serious cardiovascular events in children and young adults. *N Engl J Med*. 2011;365:1896-1904.

28 Habel LA, Cooper WO, Sox CM, et al. ADHD medications and risk of serious cardiovascular events in young and middle-aged adults. *JAMA*. 2011;306:2673-2683.

29 Michelson D, Adler L, Spencer T, et al. Atomoxetine in adults with ADHD: two randomized, placebo-controlled studies. *Biological Psychiatry*. 2003;53:112-120.

30 Adler L, Dietrich A, Reimherr FW, et al. Safety and tolerability of once versus twice daily atomoxetine in adults with ADHD. *Ann Clin Psychiatry*. 2006;18:107-113.

31 Adler LA, Spencer T, Brown TE, et al. Once-daily atomoxetine for adult attention-deficit/hyperactivity disorder: a 6-month, double-blind trial. *J Clin Psychopharmacol*. 2009;29:44-50.

32 Kemner JE, Starr HL, Ciccone PE, Hooper-Wood CG, Crockett RS. Outcomes of OROS methylphenidate compared with atomoxetine in children with ADHD: a multicenter, randomized prospective study. *Adv Ther*. 2005;22:498-512.

33 Wang Y, Zheng Y, Du Y, et al. Atomoxetine versus methylphenidate in paediatric outpatients with attention deficit hyperactivity disorder: a randomized, double-blind comparison trial. *Aust N Z J Psychiatry*. 2007;41:222-230.

34 Hazell PL, Kohn MR, Dickson R, Walton RJ, Granger RE, van Wyk GW. Core ADHD symptom improvement with atomoxetine versus methylphenidate: A direct comparison meta-analysis. *J Atten Disord*. 2010;41:335-231.

35 Summary of product characteristics: Strattera 10mg, 18mg, 25mg, 40mg, 60mg or 80mg hard capsules. www.medicines.org.uk/emc/medicine/14482/SPC/Strattera++10Umg,+18mg,+25mg,+40mg,+60mg+or+80mg+hard+capsules/. Accessed August 25, 2012.

36 Witcher JW, Long A, Smith B, et al. Atomoxetine pharmacokinetics in children and adolescent with attention deficit hyperactivity disorder. *J Child Adolesc Psychopharmacol*. 2003;13:53-63.

37 Maneeton N, Maneeton B, Srisurapanont M, Martin SD. Bupropion for adults with attention-deficit hyperactivity disorder: meta-analysis of randomized, placebo-controlled trials. *Psychiatry Clin Neurosci*. 2011;65:611-617.

38 Kim D, Steinhart B. Seizures induced by recreational abuse of bupropion tablets via nasal insufflation. *CJEM*. 2010;12:158-161.

39 Heal DJ, Cheetham SC, Smith SL. The neuropharmacology of ADHD drugs in vivo: insights on efficacy and safety. *Neuropharmacology*. 2009;57:608-618.

40 Wuo-Silva R, Fukushiro DF, Borçoi AR, et al. Addictive potential of modafinil and cross-sensitization with cocaine: a pre-clinical study. *Addict Biol*. 2011;16:565-579.

41 Bond DJ, Hadjipavlou G, Lam RW, McIntyre RS, Beaulieu S, Schaffer A, Weiss M. The Canadian Network for Mood and Anxiety Treatments (CANMAT) task force recommendations for the management of patients with mood disorders and comorbid attention-deficit/hyperactivity disorder. *Ann Clin Psychiatry.* 2012;24:23-37.

42 Findling RL, Greenhill LL, McNamara NK, et al. Venlafaxine in the treatment of children and adolescents with attention-deficit/hyperactivity disorder. *J Child Adolesc Psychopharmacol.* 2007;17:433-445.

43 Zarinara AR, Mohammadi MR, Hazrati N, et al. Venlafaxine versus methylphenidate in pediatric outpatients with attentiondeficithyperactivitydisorder: a randomized, double-blind comparison trial. *Hum Psychopharmacol.* 2010;25:530-535.

44 Agarwal V, Sitholey P. Combination of atomoxetine and methylphenidate in attention deficit/hyperactivity disorder: a case report. *J Can Acad Child Adolesc Psychiatry.* 2008;17:160.

Chapter 8

Psychological treatments

As people with attention deficit hyperactivity disorder (ADHD) mature, they often experience a gradual decline in their symptoms, although around two-thirds of cases continue to experience significant symptoms that impair functioning into their adult years [1–4]. Findings from clinical studies indicate that impulsivity and hyperactivity tend to lessen as patients reach adulthood [5,6] and problems associated with poor time management and organization become more common [7]. Nevertheless, in some cases, persisting hyperactivity and impulsive behavior can be severe.

Adults with ADHD can have many problems related to persistence of the disorder, including academic underachievement, occupational difficulties, unemployment, problems with interpersonal relationships, a sense of failure, and low self esteem. Furthermore, comorbid problems are often present, including mood and anxiety disorders, emotional lability, frustration, irritability, sleep disturbances, alcohol and substance misuse, personality disorders, antisocial behavior, and social skills deficits. Although adults with ADHD often develop effective coping strategies, many do not [8], and in the absence of such strategies, the symptoms can have a severely negative life impact [9].

A significant number of adults with ADHD presenting for treatment are newly diagnosed rather than being 'graduates' of child and adolescent services. Unfortunately, there are still many people who 'slip through the cracks' and whose ADHD has not been recognized for many years. Those who are diagnosed with ADHD in adulthood often have a history

UKAAN, *Handbook for Attention Deficit Hyperactivity*
Disorder in Adults, DOI: 10.1007/978-1-908517-79-1_8,
© Springer Healthcare 2013

of multiple presentations to child and adult services [10,11], and qualitative research has suggested that for these people psychological support is required at the time of diagnosis, to support a process of adjustment in coming to terms with their diagnosis and its prognosis [12]. This need is also recognized by their partners [13]. Psychological treatment can then shift to the treatment of skills deficits and comorbid problems. The aim is to help people so that they can better structure their daily activities and succeed in them, and to improve individual and interpersonal skills so they may achieve their potential.

Psychological treatment, in particular cognitive behavioral therapy (CBT), has strong empirical evidence for changing thoughts and beliefs that may lead to dysfunctional behavior. For people with ADHD, CBT is usually provided as a complementary treatment alongside medication. In recent years, there has been an increase in research that demonstrates the effectiveness of psychological treatments for adults with ADHD, and it seems that in many cases combined medication and CBT is more beneficial than medication alone, with significant treatment effects for symptoms of ADHD [14–20]. In comparison with a waiting-list control group, CBT and psychoeducation provided in a brief intensive group format, was found to be effective in raising self-efficacy and self esteem in adults with ADHD [21], and these are important factors for motivating treatment engagement (for a review of nonpharmacological treatments of ADHD across the lifespan, see Young and Amarasinghe [7]).

NICE clinical guidelines

There was an insufficient number of controlled studies evaluating psychological treatments in adults with ADHD for the NICE Clinical Guidelines [22] to extend the recommendations made for children into adulthood (ie, that psychological treatment should be considered a possible first-line treatment for patients with mild-to-moderate symptoms and impairments). It should be noted, however, that several studies have been reported since that time increasing the evidence base for the effectiveness of psychological interventions for ADHD in adults (reviewed in Young and Amarasinghe [7]). Even where there was a lack of direct evidence, the NICE guideline group recognized that this did not mean that psychological treatments are ineffective in adults and, indeed, considered that they may also be appropriate for those who are experiencing symptom remission. Thus, NICE made the following recommendations relating to psychological treatment for adults with ADHD:

- Drug treatment should be the first-line treatment unless the person would prefer a psychological approach.
- Drug treatment for adults with ADHD should always form part of a comprehensive treatment program that addresses psychological, behavioral, and educational or occupational needs.
- For adults with ADHD stabilized on medication but with persisting functional impairment associated with the disorder, or where there has been no response to drug treatment, a course of either group CBT or individual CBT to address the person's functional impairment should be considered. Group therapy is recommended as the first-line psychological treatment because it is the most cost-effective.
- For adults with ADHD, CBT may be considered when:
  - the person has made an informed choice not to have drug treatment;
  - drug treatment has proved to be only partially effective or ineffective or the person is intolerant to it;
  - the person has difficulty accepting the diagnosis of ADHD and accepting and adhering to drug treatment;
  - symptoms are remitting and psychological treatment is considered sufficient to target residual (mild to moderate) functional impairment.

Cognitive behavioral therapy

There is good evidence for the use of CBT both to treat symptoms and the comorbid problems seen in adults with ADHD. Randomized controlled trials (RCTs) have evaluated treatment outcome for both group and individual CBT delivery in samples that are taking ADHD medication. Most studies compare outcomes in a CBT-plus-medication group with outcomes in a medication-only 'treatment as usual' group; however, three studies include an additional control treatment in the medication-only group of supportive treatment [18], cognitive training [19], and relaxation training [17]. Individual treatment trials have shown medium-to-large treatment effects for self-rated ADHD symptom reduction [15,17,19] and informant-rated ADHD symptom reduction [15,17], with effects being maintained 1 year later [17]. Medium-to-large treatment effects have also been reported for improvement in self- and informant-rated anxiety as well as informant-rated depression symptoms [15].

Group treatments were recommended by NICE due to their likely resource and cost-efficiency. There have been a handful of RCTs to date evaluating treatment outcome for CBT delivered in groups. These have reported medium-to-large treatment effects for improvement in ADHD symptoms from self-ratings [16,18] and informant ratings [16,18,23]. In addition, post-treatment medium-to-large effects have been reported for improved organization skills [18,23], self esteem [23], anger [23], and prosocial behavior [16]. Emilsson and colleagues [16] followed up their sample 3 months later and found that the treatment effect increased over time; at follow-up they reported large treatment effects for self-rated ADHD symptoms, prosocial behavior, emotional control, anxiety, depression, informant-rated ADHD symptoms, and clinical global impression. This was supported by independent evaluations of ADHD symptoms and global functioning, which had large effect sizes. The findings suggest that those who completed a highly structured manualized CBT intervention continued to use the strategies learned in sessions after they finished treatment and therefore the treatment effect persisted and became greater over time. Similarly, Stevenson et al reported that a large treatment effect was maintained at 12-month follow-up for ADHD symptoms, organization skills, self esteem, and anger [23].

Cognitive behavioral paradigm

Young and Bramham [24] have proposed a cognitive-behavioral model of ADHD that stems from the relationship between neurocognitive deficits and early experiences (Figure 8.1). The model indicates that core symptoms (including memory problems, problem-solving difficulties, and a desire for immediate gratification) influence the ADHD child's academic achievement, behavior, mood, and social and family relationships.

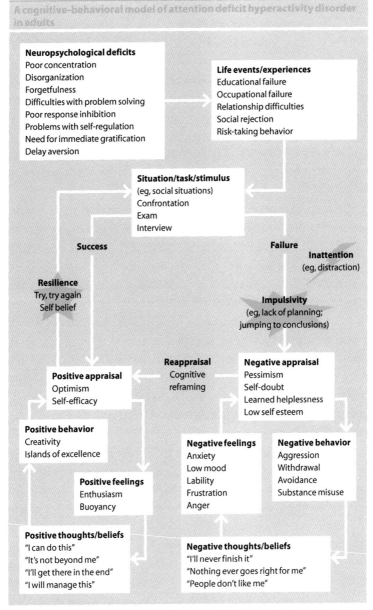

Figure 8.1 A cognitive-behavioral model of attention deficit hyperactivity disorder in adults.
ADHD, attention deficit hyperactivity disorder. Reprinted with permission from Young and Bramham [24].

However, maturity brings different problems, including difficulties with friendships and intimate relationships, occupational problems, and sometimes delinquent behavior. Not every child will have a history of failure, but most will grow up aware that, for example, they have not reached their personal potential or that they compare unfavorably with their siblings. This leads them to appraise situations negatively, to doubt their own abilities, to develop low self esteem, and to anticipate failure in their future endeavors. For many people this would normally lead to a negative cycle and self-fulfilling prophecy; however, there is some evidence that suggests that adults with ADHD tend to reappraise or cognitively reframe stressful situations [8].

It has been suggested that this strategy interrupts the negative cycle process by turning it into a motivational force that compels change [24]. This is consistent with the Drive Theory of Hull (1943) [25], which suggests that humans are driven to reduce arousal or tension in order to maintain a sense of comfort and equilibrium. This may explain the apparent resilience of people with ADHD as their tendency to engage in a process of positively reframing negative outcomes causes them to repeat their endeavours and attempts to succeed. Their resilience is characterized by the continual ability to compensate and adapt, and this most likely reflects an underlying self-efficacy. It is thus important that psychological treatment draws on this aspect of the ADHD character, since creativity and resilience are strengths that will optimize the success of psychological treatment.

NICE identified CBT to be the most appropriate intervention because it is person-centered and highly structured. The strength of CBT is its flexibility and adaptability. At times the cognitive component may be minimal or limited to one specific technique, such as coping self-talk with the predominant emphasis being on behavioral techniques. Alternatively, the therapist may shift the emphasis to include more cognitive interventions that aim to reduce psychological distress and maladaptive behavior by altering cognitive processes. Table 8.1 shows a suggested treatment outline (more information can be found from the Young–Bramham program, which provides detailed treatment plans and materials to be used in treatment for both individual and group delivery [24]).

Suggested treatment outline

1. Determine treatment goals
2. Formulate an intervention plan
3. Prioritize targets for intervention and teach the patient how to deal with procrastination
4. Provide psychoeducation about ADHD
5. CBT to address:
   - core symptoms and associated difficulties (eg, inattention, impulsivity, disorganization, time-management problems, procrastination, emotional lability)
   - comorbid problems (eg, anxiety, low mood, poor social skills, relationship problems, frustration, anger, sleep disturbance, substance misuse)
   - These treatments require adaptation as appropriate for delivery to people with ADHD
6. Monitor and evaluate progress (including analysis of obstacles to success)

Table 8.1 Suggested treatment outline. ADHD, attention deficit hyperactivity disorder; CBT, cognitive behavioral therapy.

The goals of treatment

The primary goal of treatment is to reduce symptoms or characteristics that interfere with healthy, developmentally appropriate functioning or behavior. A second goal of treatment is to improve the person's quality of life by acknowledging and treating the problems that are associated with ADHD, such as psychiatric comorbid problems, low self esteem and/or interpersonal relationship problems.

Medication may improve core symptoms and predispose the patient to benefit from psychological treatments as he or she will become more able to meet the fundamental requirements of needing to stay in the room, listen to what is being said, and collaborate with the treatment.

Psychological treatments can then teach cognitive behavioral internal strategies to improve concentration and curb impulsive behavior, and external strategies that teach the person to manipulate or adapt the environment to become one that is more optimal for success in his or her endeavors. These strategies will foster confidence and improve self-efficacy.

In order to evaluate the effectiveness of psychological treatments, outcome measures need to match the treatment goals. Specific interventions (eg, an intervention that focuses on attention and memory skills) require specific outcome measures, whereas more general indicators of outcome (eg, self esteem measures) are required for eclectic treatments.

Treatment is not just directed at the core symptoms of ADHD. Therapy sessions may include techniques that will help the patient:

- to improve emotional control;
- to self-impose structure;
- to develop organizational skills;
- to plan and manage time;
- to improve social skills and manage interpersonal relationships with peers and family;
- to improve conduct;
- to stop and think about consequences;
- to develop critical thinking and reasoning skills.

The therapist has a fair amount of licence within the treatment sessions and while one treatment may focus on one or two of these aspects, others may draw on several. What is provided must be guided by what is required, and this will often be determined by comorbid problems. Thus, unless a highly structured program is being delivered, the content and emphasis of the sessions will vary.

Psychoeducation

Providing psychoeducation about ADHD is an essential component of treatment in order to promote knowledge and understanding about the disorder and what can be expected in the years to come, and to dispel lay beliefs and/or incorrect assumptions. This education needs to include explanations about:

- the etiology of ADHD;
- ADHD symptoms;
- common psychiatric comorbidities;
- psychosocial problems;
- treatment options and side effects;
- outcome research data;
- longer-term prognosis.

It is recommended that written material should be provided to supplement discussion in sessions in order that the information can be revised later by the patient outside the sessions and/or reviewed in discussions with family members. It will also be very helpful for the patient to be directed to websites and support groups so that he or she may stay abreast of advances in the field and gain peer support.

Cognitive behavioral therapy for attention deficit hyperactivity disorder symptoms

Clinical trials suggest that impulsivity and hyperactivity tend to diminish but that attentional problems persist into adulthood [5,6], and adult symptoms are often experienced as difficulty with time management and organization. For people whose symptoms are not recognized until adolescence or later and are diagnosed de novo, psychological treatments will help them to accept their diagnosis and reframe their past experiences.

The treatment of core symptoms will involve the provision and rehearsal of coping strategies and skills development techniques, including:

- cognitive remediation strategies to address core deficits in attention, impulsivity, and emotional regulation;
- cognitive restructuring strategies that aim to change negative thought patterns;
- cognitive reframing techniques to challenge past beliefs and assumptions;
- problem-solving techniques and consequential thinking;
- setting behavioral experiments to test new skills;
- the rehearsal of adaptive behaviors.

The aim is to work with patients to generate a repertoire of practical strategies that they can successfully apply to:

- improve their attention and memory (eg, using self-instructional training and memory aids);
- develop better impulse-control skills (eg, using 'stop and think techniques'); and
- improve time-management, organizational, prioritization and planning skills (eg, by using diaries and time schedules).

Cognitive behavioral therapy for comorbid and associated problems

Most adults with ADHD have experienced a host of negative life events, including academic underachievement, occupational difficulties and unemployment, interpersonal relationship problems, and divorce. It is hardly surprising that comorbid and psychosocial problems are the rule rather than the exception, and these include mood and anxiety disorders, emotional lability, frustration, irritability, sleep disturbances, problems with alcohol and substance misuse, personality disorders (primarily cluster B), antisocial behavior, social skills deficits, poor interpersonal relationships, and a sense of failure and low self esteem.

Some generic interventions that will be helpful in treating these problems include strategies to help the patient to learn and develop protocols for problem-solving, social communication skills, self-monitoring skills, social-perspective taking, emotional control, management of lability, and assertiveness training.

The treatment of comorbid and psychosocial problems does not differ greatly from treatment that would be given to non-ADHD patients other than in their delivery. In order to optimize success, these interventions need to be adapted for patients with ADHD by:

- the delivery of individual treatment on a 'little and often' basis, for patients with severe impairments who struggle to sustain focus in a 1-hour treatment session;
- the provision of appointment reminders (by telephone, text, or email);
- the supplementation of psychoeducation, specific treatment strategies, and 'learning points' with written materials;
- the inclusion of feedback and reinforcement mechanisms that are provided on a more frequent basis;
- the introduction of reward systems (both immediate and delayed) to motivate adherence and reward achievement.

Dialectical behavioral therapy

Dialectical behavioral therapy (DBT) was developed from CBT and initially adapted to suit the specific needs of people with borderline personality disorder [26]. DBT aims to meet the needs of people with emotional problems by encouraging them to dialectically balance acceptance with change, hence CBT techniques to change behavior are supplemented with 'acceptance strategies' that focus on validation. A RCT evaluating DBT in comparison to an unstructured discussion group (all patients being on ADHD medication) has reported a medium post-treatment effect for improvement in ADHD symptoms but no statistically significant differences in measures of anxiety, depression, sleep, and stress [20].

Coaching

Coaching is a growing area in the management of ADHD and this supportive intervention generally applies a brief, solution-focused paradigm. It should be noted that coaching does not draw on any clear methodology and that, in general, coaches are not required to have any specific qualifications. Nevertheless, there are reports that suggest that coaching is a helpful supplement to group CBT ADHD interventions [16,23] and may improve completion rates [27], possibly reflecting that individual coaching sessions support participants to transfer skills learned in the process of treatment and apply them into their daily lives.

Coaching has been utilized in two key ways:

- to support group CBT treatments with the aim of improving completion rates and the transference of skills from a therapeutic 'theoretical' setting to an existential setting;
- to facilitate individual performance.

These aims are achieved by the coach adopting a tutoring or instructional approach within a collaborative partnership that aims to provide structure, support, and feedback. The intervention draws on patients' personal strengths and helps them to better manage their lives through mentoring and supporting them to set and achieve goals in their daily activities. This also involves the development of functioning problem-solving skills and coping strategies. The work to be undertaken is most commonly negotiated on an individual basis between coach and client but essentially focuses on the client's goals and needs. Since there is no standard methodology, the process of the intervention varies considerably; it may include face-to-face contact, brief regular telephone conversations, text messaging, and email contact [7]. One CBT intervention, the R&R2 for ADHD Youths and Adults, includes structured coaching sessions to supplement the group treatment [16,28].

Summary

As adolescents move into adulthood, they increasingly face responsibility for structuring and managing their own time and activities [4]. For those with ADHD, psychological support and treatment is warranted [7]. Those with comorbid psychiatric conditions and adults who have been newly diagnosed as having ADHD may need more intensive psychological treatment.

NICE guidelines state that drug treatment should be considered the first-line therapy for adults with ADHD unless the person would prefer a psychological approach [22]. However, the NICE guidelines note that, despite the lack of a strong evidence base for the use of psychological therapies in ADHD, their effectiveness is not in doubt and, moreover, they emphasize that there is a need to provide comprehensive programs to address psychological, behavioral, and occupational problems. The guidelines also recommend that for those whose symptoms are decreasing in severity, psychological therapies may be sufficient to manage residual functional impairments. CBT is likely to be the most appropriate intervention because of its highly structured and person-centered nature. Group treatments are likely to be the most resourceful and cost-effective.

References

1   McCarthy S, Asherson P, Coghill D, et al. Attention-deficit hyperactivity disorder: treatment discontinuation in adolescents and young adults. *Br J Psychiatry*. 2009;194:273-277.

2   Faraone SV, Biederman J, Mick E. The age-dependent decline of attention deficit hyperactivity disorder: a meta-analysis of follow-up studies. *Psychol Med*. 2006;36:159-165.

3   Young S, Gudjonsson G. Growing out of attention-deficit/hyperactivity disorder: the relationship between functioning and symptoms. *J Atten Disord*. 2008;12:162-169.

4   Young S, Murphy CM, Coghill D. Avoiding the 'twilight zone': Guidance and recommendations on ADHD and the transition between child and adult services. *BMC Psychiatry*. 2011;11:174.

5   Biederman J, Mick E, Faraone SV. Age-dependent decline of symptoms of attention deficit hyperactivity disorder: impact of remission definition and symptom type. *Am J Psychiatry*. 2000;157:816-818.

6   Ingram S, Hechtman L, Morgenstern G. Outcome issues in ADHD: adolescent and adult long-term outcome. *Ment Retard Dev Disabil Res Rev*. 1999;5:243-250.

7   Young S, Amarasinghe JA. Practitioner Review: non-pharmacological treatments for ADHD: A lifespan approach. *J Child Psychol Psychiatry*. 2010;51:116-133.

8   Young S. Coping strategies used by ADHD adults. *Pers Individ Dif*. 2005;38:809-816.

9   Wender P. *Attention Deficit Hyperactivity Disorder in Children and Adults*. New York: Oxford University Press; 2000.

10 Dalsgaard S, Mortensen PB, Frydenberg M, et al. Conduct problems, gender and the adult psychiatric outcome of children with attention-deficit hyperactivity disorder. *Br J Psychiatry*. 2002;181:416-421.

11 Young S, Toone B, Tyson C. Comorbidity and psychosocial profile of adults with attention deficit hyperactivity disorder. *Pers Individ Dif*. 2003;35:743-755.

12 Young S, Bramham J, Gray K, Rose E. The experience of receiving a diagnosis and treatment of ADHD in adulthood: a qualitative study of clinically referred patients using Interpretative Phenomenological Analysis. *J Atten Disord*. 2008;11:493-503.

13 Young S, Gray K, Bramham J. A phenomenological analysis of the experience of receiving a diagnosis and treatment of ADHD in adulthood: a partner's perspective. *J Atten Disord*. 2009;12:299-307.

14 Rostain AL, Ramsay JR. A combined treatment approach for adults with ADHD - results of an open study of 43 patients. *J Atten Disord*. 2006;10:150-159.

15 Safren SA, Otto MW, Sprich S, et al. Cognitive-behavioral therapy for ADHD in medication-treated adults with continued symptoms. *Behav Res Ther*. 2005;43:831-842.

16 Emilsson B, Gudjonsson G, Sigurdsson JF, et al. Cognitive behavior therapy in medication-treated adults with ADHD and persistent symptoms: a randomized controlled trial. *BMC Psychiatry*. 2011;11:116-125.

17 Safren SA, Sprich S, Mimiaga MJ, et al. Cognitive behavioral therapy vs relaxation with educational support for medication-treated adults with ADHD and persistent symptoms: a randomized controlled trial. *JAMA*. 2010;304:875-880.

18 Solanto MV, Marks DJ, Wasserstein J, et al. Efficacy of meta-cognitive therapy for adult ADHD. *Am J Psychiatry*. 2010;167:958-968.

19 Virta M, Salakari A, Antila M, et al. Short cognitive behavioral therapy and cognitive training for adults with ADHD – a randomized controlled pilot study. *Neuropsychiatr Dis Treat*. 2010;10:443-453.

20 Hirvikoski T, Waaler E, Alfredsson J, et al. Reduced ADHD symptoms in adults with ADHD after structured skills training group: Results from a randomized controlled trial. *Behav Res Ther*. 2011;49:175-185.

21 Bramham J, Young S, Bickerdike A, et al. Evaluation of group cognitive behavioral therapy for adults with ADHD. *J Atten Disord*. 2009;12:434-441.

22 National Institute for Health and Clinical Excellence (NICE). Attention Deficit Hyperactivity Disorder: Diagnosis and Management of ADHD in Children, Young People and Adults. NICE Clinical Guideline 72.; NICE website. 2009. www.nice.org.uk/CG72. Accessed August 25, 2012.

23 Stevenson CS, Whitmont S, Bornholt L, et al. A cognitive remediation program for adults with attention deficit hyperactivity disorder. *Aust N Z J Psychiatry*. 2002;36:610-616.

24 Young S, Bramham J. *Cognitive Behavoiural Therapy for ADHD in Adolescents and Adults: A Psychological Guide to Practice*. Chichester: John Wiley and Sons Ltd; 2012.

25 Hull CL. *Principles of Behavior*. New York: Appleton-Century-Crofts; 1943.

26 Linehan MM. Dialectical behavior therapy for treatment of borderline personality disorder: implications for the treatment of substance abuse. *NIDA Research Monographs*. 1993;137:201-215.

27 Hollin CR, Palmer EJ. Offending behavior programmes: controversies and resolutions. In: Holin CJ, Palmer EJ, eds. *Offending Behavior Programmes: Development, Application and Controversies*. Chichester: John Wiley and Sons; 2006.

28 Young SJ, Ross RR. *R&R2 for ADHD youths and adults. A Prosocial Competence Training Program*. Ottawa: Cognitive Centre of Canada; 2007.

Chapter 9

Attention deficit hyperactivity disorder during pregnancy

Current research indicates a strong familial risk for the development of attention deficit hyperactivity disorder (ADHD) among offspring of parents with ADHD that results from genetic risk factors (see Chapter 3). The rate of ADHD among first-degree relatives is reported to be in the region of 10–20% for the siblings and parents of a child with ADHD [1,2]. However, the genetic transmission is complex and not sufficiently understood to enable clinicians to offer any specific prenatal advice to mothers with ADHD. Though genes play a part in the development of the disorder, it is clear that social, educational, and psychological factors also play an impor tant role in developmental course and long-term outcome, and therefore genetic loading should not be seen as the only determining factor. General advice should therefore be given to parents with ADHD on the risk to their offspring of developing ADHD, and strategies considered to reduce any potentially negative effects of parental ADHD on their developing child.

Overall, there is no evidence that parental ADHD per se has a negative impact on pregnancy. Many mothers with ADHD manage to cope with all aspects of pregnancy and parenthood; in other cases, as with all patients with ADHD, there may be potentially detrimental problems such as high levels of stress, poor self-care, and the use of alcohol, tobacco, and/or drugs. There are two main considerations when it comes to ADHD and pregnancy:

- the decision whether or not to continue drug treatment for ADHD during pregnancy (or when expecting a pregnancy);
- the impact of maternal behavior during pregnancy on the future child.

UKAAN, *Handbook for Attention Deficit Hyperactivity Disorder in Adults*, DOI: 10.1007/978-1-908517-79-1_9, © Springer Healthcare 2013

General considerations

Although it is unlikely that treatment with ADHD medication will be initiated in a pregnant patient, it remains to be considered what to do if a patient who is already receiving psychopharmacological treatment becomes pregnant. In such cases, it is essential to consider the possible benefits and risks of treatment before deciding whether or not to discontinue medication. Each case has to be assessed individually since there are a range of possible outcomes. The decision-making process depends on several factors including:

- risk for the developing baby from detrimental maternal behavior or maternal stress during the pregnancy;
- efficacy of the present treatment and its side effects;
- the nature and severity of the ADHD symptoms and the impact of medication on controlling these and associated comorbidities;
- individual circumstances including social support and adjustment, engagement with health care professionals (eg, midwife, health visitor) and self-care during the pregnancy.

Treatment

Both treatment and nontreatment bear risks. While discontinuation of medication reduces the risk of chemically harming the child, it may lead to an increase in potentially harmful behaviors related to the mother's mental state. There may be a general deterioration in the mother's mental health, including erratic and disorganized behavior and poor risk management (such as dangerous driving or the use of drugs, alcohol, or tobacco during pregnancy). Impulsive behavior, carelessness, and emotional instability are all associated with ADHD in adults. Risk to the developing baby may also arise from increased stress levels.

Exposure to pharmacological agents

Available data relating to the risk of prenatal exposure to stimulant medication is limited. Amphetamines, methylphenidate, atomoxetine, bupropion, and modafinil are all designated category C by the FDA. This category includes drugs where animal studies have reported some harm without there being any robust evidence in humans, or where no human or animal studies have been performed.

Methylphenidate and dexamphetamine: There are few data available regarding the risk of prenatal exposure to these drugs. At therapeutic doses, there does not seem to be an increased rate of fetal malformations. However, it has been well-established that illicit use of stimulants is associated with prematurity, low birth weight, and increased morbidity both in the mother and child [3].

Atomoxetine: The data relating to atomoxetine are even more limited. In single cases of atomoxetine use during pregnancy, no teratogenicity was reported. However, in animal models, atomoxetine exposure, at least in high doses, can result in negative effects, including decreased survival rates, lower birth weight, delayed ossification, and abnormal angiogenesis [3].

Other drug treatments: A higher incidence of cardiac abnormalities has been reported with bupropion, though a recent study in a large US cohort failed to show any increased risk when compared with other antidepressants [4]. There are no adequate studies of modafinil in pregnancy that allow an evaluation of its teratogenic potential. If an informed decision is made to continue drug treatment during pregnancy, some general rules are advisable:

- Adjust dosage to the minimum amount that produces good control of symptoms. During pregnancy both volume of distribution and liver enzymatic activity are increased. This may result in less active drug being available, which makes reduction of dosage challenging. However, some women report spontaneous improvement in attentional symptoms during pregnancy, and in these patients a dose reduction may be easier to achieve.
- Titrate down or stop stimulant dosage prior to delivery to avoid the potential for acute withdrawal symptoms in the newborn.
- Liaise closely with the obstetric team and provide full information on treatment.
- Increase frequency of follow-ups to assess changes in mental state during pregnancy and in the postpartum period.

Maternal behavior during pregnancy

Maternal factors that have been associated with an increased risk of ADHD include:

- exposure to nicotine in utero [5,6];
- alcohol use during pregnancy [7];
- maternal caffeine intake [5];
- exposure to psychosocial stress [7,8].

Although smoking during pregnancy has been widely discussed as a risk factor for the later development of ADHD, it is not clear that this is a direct toxic effect of smoking. Rather, recent studies suggest that the association between mothers smoking during pregnancy and offspring ADHD is not causal, but reflects genetic effects being passed down from the mother to the child [9]. Nevertheless, smoking has other detrimental effects on the developing fetus and should be avoided. Data regarding the possible risk of caffeine exposure are weak and are not convincing [5].

The evidence that maternal stress exposure during pregnancy increases rates of offspring ADHD is more consistent, and the level of maternal stress is reported to be associated with the severity of ADHD symptoms among offspring [6]. Stress exposure is a risk factor that is independent of maternal smoking, although stress and maternal smoking are thought to be closely related [8].

Low birth weight and prematurity are both associated with development of ADHD [10–12]. More generally, complications during pregnancy, delivery, and infancy may contribute to an increased risk of ADHD independently of possible genetic factors. Pregnancy risks may be greatest for complications of a chronic nature such as, family psychosocial problems, and illicit drug use. Furthermore, such complications are also associated with impaired cognitive functioning and poor school performance, both of which are associated with ADHD [13].

The lack of information on the risks to offspring from exposure to ADHD drug treatments leads to the general recommendation that treatments for ADHD during pregnancy should be considered individually and decided once all risks are considered and the patient has been fully informed. This should be balanced against the severity of ADHD in the mother and the effectiveness of the drugs to control detrimental behaviors that could also put the developing child at risk. Increased stress, low birth weight, prematurity, and the use of drugs and/or alcohol during pregnancy are common risk factors to fetal development that could increase if medication for ADHD is stopped during pregnancy and should therefore be taken into account.

In summary, the treatment of ADHD during pregnancy should be decided on a case-by-case basis, considering the severity of symptoms, comorbidities, risks, and support available for the individual patient. It should be remembered that both continuing drug treatment and stopping treatment have risks. Psychological therapies should be considered in these patients as described in Chapter 7.

Attention deficit hyperactivity disorder treatment and breastfeeding

All psychotropic drugs are excreted through breast milk. In general, the concentration of drugs in breast milk is around 1% of that in blood. In general, if a child has been exposed to a psychotropic drug in utero, it will not be necessary to stop medication during breastfeeding as the amount it will receive through breast milk will be inferior to the exposure during pregnancy. Ideally, the prescribed medication should be given as a once-a-day formulation and before the child's longest period of sleep to avoid a feed occurring during the peak secretion period. Drugs that are licensed for use in children are in general less risky than those that have not been tested in children. If medication is used at the same time as breastfeeding, potential effects of the drug on the child's development should be monitored and the child's pediatrician should be informed of any changes in medication dosage or formulation.

In relation to the specific effects of stimulant and nonstimulant medication that reach the child through breastfeeding, little is known. Some case reports suggest that methylphenidate is relatively innocuous, particularly if given after the morning feed but there is very little evidence about any longer term effects [14]. Caution should be exercised with atomoxetine and amphetamines. Modafinil is contraindicated in women who are breastfeeding [15]. Bupropion accumulates in breast milk and increases the risk of seizures in the newborn [16].

The postnatal period is a stressful and challenging time for women with ADHD. A great deal of organization and planning is required to meet the demands of a new child. Many women with ADHD will request to be restarted on medication after delivery. In this case, risks and benefits need to be carefully considered and a decision on whether to restart medication or whether to continue breastfeeding should be reached on an individual basis. In most cases, breastfeeding should not be continued when taking psychotropic medications.

References

1   Chen W, Zhou K, Sham P, et al. DSM-IV combined type ADHD shows familial association with sibling trait scores: a sampling strategy for QTL linkage. *Am J Med Genet B Neuropsychiatr Genet*. 2008;147B:1450-1460.

2   Faraone SV, Biederman J, Monuteaux MC. Toward guidelines for pedigree selection in genetic studies of attention deficit hyperactivity disorder. *Genet Epidemiol*. 2000;18:1-16.

3   Humphreys C, Garcia-Bournissen F, Ito S, et al. Exposure to attention deficit hyperactivity disorder medications during pregnancy. *Can Fam Phys*. 2007;53:1153-1155.

4   Cole JA, Modell JG, Haight BR, Cosmatos IS, Stoler JM, Walker AM. Bupropion in pregnancy and the prevalence of congenital malformations. *Pharmacoepidemiol Drug Saf*. 2007;16:474-484.

5   Linnet KM, Dalsgaard S, Obel C, et al. Maternal lifestyle factors in pregnancy risk of attention deficit hyperactivity disorder and associated behaviors: review of the current evidence. *Am J Psychiatry*. 2003;160:1028-1040.

6   Rodriguez A, Bohlin G. Are maternal smoking and stress during pregnancy related to ADHD symptoms in children? *J Child Psychol Psychiatry*. 2005;46:246-254.

7   de Zeeuw P, Zwart F, Schrama R, van Engeland H, Durston S. Prenatal exposure to cigarette smoke or alcohol and cerebellum volume in attention-deficit/hyperactivity disorder and typical development. *Transl Psychiatry*. 2012;2:e84.

8   Grizenko N, Shayan YR, Polotskaia A, et al. Relation of maternal stress during pregnancy to symptom severity and response to treatment in children with ADHD. *J Psychiatr Neurosci*. 2008; 33:10-16.

9   Thapar A, Rice F, Hay D, et al. Prenatal smoking might not cause attention-deficit/hyperactivity disorder: evidence from a novel design. *Biol Psychiatry*. 2009;66:722-727.

10 Aarnoudse-Moens CS, Weisglas-Kuperus N, van Goudoever JB, et al. Meta-analysis of neurobehavioral outcomes in very preterm and/or very low birth weight children. *Pediatrics*. 2009;124:717-728.

11 Dahl LB, Kaaresen P, Tunby J, et al. Emotional, behavioral, social, and academic outcomes in adolescents born with very low birth weight. *Pediatrics*. 2006;118:e449-e459.

12 Shum D, Neulinger K, O'Callaghan M, et al. Attentional problems in children born very preterm or with extremely low birth weight at 7–9 years. *Arch Clin Neuropsychol*. 2008;23:103-112.

13 Milberger S, Biederman J, Faraone SV, et al. Pregnancy, delivery and infancy complications and attention deficit hyperactivity disorder: issues of gene-environment interaction. *Biol Psychiatry*. 1997; 41:65-75.

14 Hackett P, Kristensen JH, Hale TW, Paterson R, Ilett KF. Methylphenidate and breast-feeding. *Pharmacother*. 2006;40:1890-1891.

15 European Medicines Agency (EMA). Modafinil summary of product characteristics. EMA website. www.ema.europa.eu/docs/en_GB/document_library/Referrals_document/ Modafinil_31/WC500099178.pdf. Accessed August 24, 2012.

16 Taddio A, Ito S. Drugs and breastfeeding. In: Koren G, ed. *Maternal-Fetal Toxicology, A Clinician's Guide*. 3rd edition. New York, US: Dekker M, Inc; 2001: 177-233.

Chapter 10

Attention deficit hyperactivity disorder and the criminal justice system

Attention deficit hyperactivity disorder and crime

The age-dependent decline of attention deficit hyperactivity disorder (ADHD) symptoms suggests that by young adulthood the full diagnosis will persist in around 15% of cases and a further 50% will be in partial remission [1]. Thus many individuals, although within the subthreshold of the *Diagnostic and Statistical Manual of Mental Disorders (DSM-IV)* criteria, still experience functional impairment due to the persistence of ADHD symptoms. The trajectory for some is a progression of comorbid conduct problems into antisocial and criminal behavior. Those who were diagnosed and treated in childhood may have better outcomes than those who did not have this advantage.

International studies suggest that a high proportion of youths (up to two-thirds) and young adults (up to half) detained in prison screen positive for ADHD [2]. This has been associated with early onset of criminal behavior, even prior to age 11 years, and high rates of recidivism. Rates in female prisoners are reported to be lower at around 10% (for a review, see Young et al [2]). In the UK, a study conducted in personality disorder wards in forensic mental health services has also reported elevated screening rates of ADHD (around one-third) [3]. UK prison studies using screening questionnaires found rates of 43% in 14-year-old youths [4] and 14% in adults [5]. All these studies have limitations in their methodologies; nevertheless, it seems that the rates of youths and

UKAAN, *Handbook for Attention Deficit Hyperactivity Disorder in Adults*, DOI: 10.1007/978-1-908517-79-1_10,
© Springer Healthcare 2013

adults with ADHD in forensic settings far exceed those reported in the general population.

The link between ADHD and crime is likely to be associated with ADHD symptoms and personality factors that are associated with their symptoms: recklessness and risk taking; sensation seeking behavior; poor behavioral control; absentmindedness or forgetfulness; compliant personality traits; labile temperament; and a confrontational interpersonal style. These young people are vulnerable and they are often disadvantaged at several stages in their interface with the criminal justice system; for example, as a suspect, witness, or defendant and post-conviction as a prison inmate or under the supervision of probation services. Chronic substance misuse among the most prolific offenders is of major concern [6] and this has been associated with both ADHD symptoms and the motivation behind offending [7]. The vulnerabilities of people with ADHD are often not recognized, which means that these individuals lack the protection that they require. Engagement within the criminal justice system is a demanding and stressful process and existing cognitive limitations are likely to be exacerbated, resulting in the individual experiencing further impairment in their attention, emotional, and behavioral control.

Experts are increasingly being asked to write reports to advise the court on the vulnerabilities and/or management of youths and adults with ADHD. Some of the key issues are summarized within this chapter (for a more detailed review, see [8]).

Vulnerability in police interviews

Individuals with ADHD may be at risk of making admissions or giving factually incorrect information during police interviews for several reasons, including maladaptive coping strategies, a desire for immediate gratification, and attention and memory problems. Their symptoms of restlessness and impulsiveness may lead them to be highly motivated to escape the confinement of custody. They may not pay full attention in the police interview, which may require that they concentrate for long periods of time and attend to important information presented both verbally and visually (eg, exhibits) at the same time as having to cope with interrogative pressure. One coping mechanism may be to resort to responding with 'don't know' responses, even for questions posed for which they should know the answer [9].

This may result in the police suspecting they are not cooperating fully with the interview process. They may be perceived as being evasive or deliberately misleading, especially as they may unintentionally provide the police with misleading accounts of events. This may be due to them not fully understanding the significance of the questions put to them or the implications of their answers. Importantly, suspects with ADHD symptoms questioned by police are at elevated risk of giving a false confession even after controlling for gender, age, emotional lability, and conduct disorder [10,11]. This suggests that their resilience to resisting pressure from police and peers is weakened by their ADHD condition rather than their false confession principally representing irresponsible and delinquent behavior associated with conduct disorder.

Ironically, in certain circumstances youths may be disadvantaged by the presence of an appropriate adult, whose primary role is to give advice to all relevant parties, to further communication, and ensure that the interview is conducted in a fair way. This person is likely to be a parent [12], and, given the strong genetic link with ADHD [13], this may be a parent with (undiagnosed) residual ADHD who will also struggle with the interview process and encourage the child to agree or 'own up' so that they can get out of the police station and go home.

Fitness to plead and stand trial

In England and Wales, the criteria for fitness to plead and stand trial (R v Pritchard, [1836] 7 C. & P. 303) requires that the defendant must be able to comprehend the proceedings of the trial; be able to challenge a juror to whom he might wish to object; understand the details of the evidence; instruct counsel; follow proceedings; and give evidence. This means that the individual has to sustain concentration, listen to what is being said, and follow the trial proceedings. The legal precedent in England and Wales was the case of Billy Jo Friend, who successfully appealed his conviction of murder because it was deemed that at the time he was unlikely to have been fit to plead and stand trial due to his severe ADHD symptoms [14].

It is not suggested that people with ADHD are not fit to plead and stand trial. In most cases, it is only necessary to recommend that special considerations are adopted by the courts, (eg, the provision of brief regular breaks, that counsel pose one question at a time and avoid using complex language). Emotional lability may be a particular problem when testifying as they may become distressed and/or angry under cross examination. Unless these vulnerabilities are explained, they are likely to be misinterpreted by a jury.

Criminal responsibility and mitigation of sentence

Mens rea refers to the defendant's state of mind at the time of the alleged offence and court assessments may be commissioned to establish whether the diagnosis of ADHD has relevance to an offence (ie, to negate criminal responsibility and/or to mitigate punishment). The legal issues relate to:

- *Intent:* the planning and desire to perform an act. People with ADHD will most likely have the ability to form intent but the key issue may relate more to recklessness (eg, carelessness). Recklessness shows less culpability than intention.
- *Duress and coercion:* knowledge of the wrongfulness of the act but robbed of free will by a perceived threat.
- *Provocation:* knowledge of the wrongfulness of the act but robbed of self-control. In law, there are two types of provocation: one is instantaneous and the other accumulative over time. The key concept of both relates to behavioral control. Individuals with ADHD may be vulnerable due to their poor emotional regulation expressed by a labile, reactive temperament and susceptibility to losing behavioral control.
- *Diminished responsibility:* 'malice aforethought' (ie, intention to kill another person or inflict grievous bodily harm). This involves the question of mitigating circumstances that may reduce the charge of murder to manslaughter. Importantly, one has to demonstrate 'substantial impairment' in perception, judgment, or willingness and this has been argued successfully in cases of depression, psychosis and personality disorder. For people with ADHD, an important issue here relates to impulsiveness and planning deficits

(ie, a tendency to act on the spur of the moment and without considering the consequences of action).

People with ADHD may be vulnerable due to their symptoms at each of the above mitigants of criminal responsibility. The extent to which their symptoms affect them will depend on the severity of their symptoms, whether they are taking prescribed ADHD medication and, if so, whether they take it regularly and the extent to which this medication is effective in treating their symptoms [15].

Post-conviction

Although it is the association with conduct disorder that may be the key vulnerability for ADHD youths and adults to become involved in crime [15], it is their ADHD symptoms that may keep them longer in the system by reducing the likelihood of early release, perhaps due to an association with aggressive incidents [3,8,16]. For example, Young et al [5] investigated the relationship between ADHD symptoms and critical incidents in 198 serving prisoners within a Scottish prison. Behavioral problems in prison were determined using a measure of recorded critical incidents over a period of 3 months, including verbal and physical aggression, damage to property, and self-injury. Functional impairment was determined by extreme frequency of critical incidents (ie, the top 10%). After controlling for antisocial personality disorder in symptomatic prisoners, including those in partial remission, ADHD symptoms accounted for a sixfold greater number of critical incidents. Institutional aggression may arise not only from poor behavioral control but also from emotional lability and dysregulation [17] and this may be magnified when coping with stressful situations. The findings indicate the importance of identifying and treating prisoners with ADHD.

Treatment of offenders with attention deficit hyperactivity disorder

With respect to their ADHD symptoms, offenders with ADHD are unlikely to differ greatly in their response to treatment with medication than nonoffenders with ADHD. A Swedish randomized controlled trial reported large treatment effects for stimulant medication in prisoners; however, the effect on behavioral outcomes has yet to be investigated in this popu-lation. The needs of these individuals are complex as they often present with multiple problems including ADHD, comorbid psychopathology, substance misuse, and personality disorder, as well as having entrenched criminal attitudes and thinking patterns. Hence, to successfully rehabili-tate offenders with ADHD, comprehensive intervention programs that map closely to their needs and reduce risk are required.

One such program is the pro-social competence program, R&R2 for ADHD Youths and Adults [18]. This program has shown large treatment effects for ADHD symptoms, pro-social behavior, emotional control, anxiety, depression, and clinical global impression when delivered to patients receiving ADHD medication in the community [19] and medium treatment effects for problem-solving, emotional stability, ADHD symp-toms, violent attitudes, and anger problems when delivered to incarcer-ated personality-disordered offenders who were not receiving ADHD medication [20].

Summary

The interface between ADHD and the criminal justice system is only just starting to be understood. The problem is that, in spite of ADHD being a common disorder in these individuals (and for which there are NICE guidelines for assessment and treatment), this condition is not 'on the radar' of criminal justice agencies and the implications for ADHD being missed or misdiagnosed are not therefore considered. Hence, psychoeducation, training, and screening materials need to be developed and implemented to resolve what appears to be a gap in knowledge and skills. The key questions for this population include:

- Will multi-modal treatment be effective in reducing institutional disruptive and violent behavior within the prison setting?
- Will it mean that individuals will engage better in educational, occupational, and therapeutic prison programs?
- Will this lead to a reduction in recidivism?

There is a pressing need for research to answer these important questions as, aside from conferring health gain to the individual and reducing risk in society, there may be important and pragmatic benefits to the justice system.

References

1   Faraone SV, Biederman J, Mick E. The age-dependent decline of attention deficit hyperactivity disorder: a meta-analysis of follow-up studies. *Psych Med*. 2006;36:159-165.

2   Young S, Adamou M, Bolea B, Gudjonsson G, Müller U, Pitts M, Thome J, Asherson P. The identification and management of ADHD offenders within the criminal justice system: a consensus statement from the UK Adult ADHD Network and criminal justice agencies. *BMC Psychiatry*. 2011;11:116.

3   Young S, Gudjonsson G, Ball S, Lam J. Attention deficit hyperactivity disorder in personality disordered offenders and the association with disruptive behavioral problems. *J Forens Psychiatry Psychol*. 2003;14:491-505.

4   Young S, Gudjonsson GH, Misch P, et al. Prevalence of ADHD symptoms among youth in a secure facility: The consistency and accuracy of self- and informant-report ratings. *J Forens Psychiatry Psychol*. 2010;21:238-246.

5   Young S, Gudjonsson GH, Wells J, et al. Attention Deficit Hyperactivity Disorder and critical incidents in a Scottish prison population. *Pers Individ Dif*. 2009;46:265-269.

6   Young S, Wells J, Gudjonsson GH. Predictors of offending among prisoners: the role of attention deficit hyperactivity disorder (ADHD) and substance use. *J Psychopharmacol*. 2011;25:1524-1532.

7   Gudjonsson GH, Wells J, Young S. Motivation for offending among prisoners and the relationship with Axis I and Axis II disorders and ADHD symptoms. *Per Individ Dif*. 2011;50:64-68.

8   Young S. Attention Deficit Hyperactivity Disorder. In, Young S, Kopelman M, Gudjonsson G. (eds), *Forensic Neuropsychology In Practice: A Guide to Assessment and Legal Processes*. New York: Oxford University Press; 2009: 81-107.

9   Gudjonsson GH, Young S, Bramham J. Interrogative suggestibility in adults diagnosed with attention-deficit hyperactivity disorder (ADHD). A potential vulnerability during police questioning. *Pers Individ Dif*. 2007;43:737-745.

10 Gudjonsson GH, Sigurdsson JF, Einarsson E, Bragason OO, Newton AK. Interrogative suggestibility, compliance and false confessions among prison inmates and their relationship with attention deficit hyperactivity disorder. *Psychol Med*. 2008;38:1037-1044.

11 Gudjonsson GH, Sigurdsson JF, Sigfusdottir ID, Young S. False confessions to police and their relationship with conduct disorder, ADHD, and life adversity *Pers Individ Dif*. 2012;52:696-701.

12 Medford S, Gudjonsson GH, Pearse J. The efficacy of the appropriate adult safeguard during police interviewing. *Leg Criminol Psychol*. 2003;8:253-266.

13 Williams NM, Zaharieva I, Martin A, et al. Rare chromosomal deletions and duplications in attention-deficit hyperactivity disorder: a genome-wide analysis. *Lancet*. 376:1401-1408.

14 Gudjonsson G, Young, S. An overlooked vulnerability in a defendant: attention deficit hyperactivity disorder (ADHD) and a miscarriage of justice. *Leg Criminol Psychol*. 2006;11:211-218.

15 Gudjonsson GH, Sigurdsson JF, Sigfusdottir ID, Young S. A national epidemiological study of offending and its relationship with ADHD symptoms and associated risk factors. *J Atten Disord*. In press.

16 Young S, Misch P, Collins P, Gudjonsson GH. Predictors of institutional behavioural disturbance and offending in the community among young offenders. *J Forens Psychiatry Psychol*. 2011;22:72-86.

17 Gudjonsson GH, Sigurdsson JF, Adalssteinsson T, Young S. The relationship between ADHD symptoms, mood instability, and self-reported offending. *J Atten Disord*. In press.

18 Young SJ, Ross RR. R&R2 for Youths and Adults with Mental Health Problems: A Prosocial Competence Training Program. Ottawa: Cognitive Centre of Canada; 2007.

19 Emilsson B, Gudjonsson G, Sigurdsson JF, et al. Cognitive behavior therapy in medication-treated adults with ADHD and persistent symptoms: a randomized controlled trial. *BMC Psychiatry*. 2011;11:116-125.

20 Young S, Hopkin G, Perkins D, Farr C, Doidge A, Gudjonsson GH. A controlled trial of a cognitive skills program for personality disordered offenders. *J Atten Disord*. In press.

Chapter 11

Service provision for adults with attention deficit hyperactivity disorder

To be able to access an attention deficit hyperactivity disorder (ADHD) service, patients follow a number of pathways. Clinical care pathways for mental health vary according to country, and for the UK have been described since the 1980s [1]. For children with ADHD, these have been revisited more recently [2] but these pathways have yet to be adequately examined for adults. This lack of evidence base has implications for developing models for service delivery for adults with ADHD.

The whole of the scientific literature that examines the development of services for people with ADHD is not vast. It started in earnest with the new millennium and focuses almost entirely on children and adolescent populations, with contributions from adult populations being rare, of small scale and poor quality. As far as the UK is concerned, the contribution to the literature is small, with only a handful of studies describing small data sets [3–6]. A recent study in the UK using a larger sample reported on trends in recognition and service use for children with ADHD [7]. The prevailing themes these studies attempted to address are as follows:

- Who seeks a service?
- What is the cost of ADHD?
- What are the trends in service delivery and service models?
- What are the local experiences and reports?

A critical summary of these themes will be discussed in this chapter.

UKAAN, *Handbook for Attention Deficit Hyperactivity Disorder in Adults*, DOI: 10.1007/978-1-908517-79-1_11, © Springer Healthcare 2013

Service populations

Most information about the profile of people who seek a clinical service for ADHD comes from child and adolescent studies. Currently, there is no UK study that provides an analysis of the different pathways based on 'disease conditions' or specific patient profiles for adults with ADHD. What currently exists is a description of the source of referrals to a few adult clinics; information that is not readily generalized within or between countries.

In the US, Hoagwood [8] summarized the evidence base in a number of areas: treatment services for children and adolescents, trends in services, types of services provided, service mix, and barriers to care. This study identified major gaps between the research evidence base and clinical practice.

Gender: Prevalence estimates converge to indicate a 3:1 ratio of boys to girls in the assignment of ADHD diagnoses [9–11]. A similar ratio of 2:1 or 3:1 (boys to girls) has also been reported for prescription of psychotropic medications [12] and methylphenidate [3]. However, in the use of specialist mental health services, the opposite finding has been reported: girls who are diagnosed with ADHD are twice as likely to use specialist mental health services as boys with this diagnosis, whereas boys are three times as likely to use pediatric services as girls [9]. Furthermore, fewer girls than boys are referred for ADHD treatment, but once they are seen, they have a similar pattern of impairment and receive similar treatment at assessment [13]. These findings suggest that there are specific gender differences in the referral pathways of children with ADHD, which could also be reflected in an adult service.

Ethnicity: Differences in ethnic groups accessing clinical services have also been noted, although few studies have sufficient sample sizes to adequately analyze such differences. In a population survey of a rural service use (the Great Smoky Mountain Study), Caucasian youths meeting the diagnostic criteria for ADHD were significantly more likely to use general medical services and twice as likely to use specialist mental health services than African-American youths [9]. This may arise because Caucasians could more easily access these services, for a number of reasons. Studies in the US have found that minority youths, primarily

African American, are less than half as likely as Caucasian youths to have been prescribed psychotropic medications [11,14,15]. Ethnicity differences have also been reported in prescriptions of psychotropic medications among Medicaid patients, with African-American youths less than half as likely as Caucasian youths to have been prescribed psychotropic medications [15]. There is no UK study addressing ethnic group differences in the treatment of ADHD.

Parental burden: The parents of children with ADHD have been studied [16] and found to have high levels of caregiver strain and low levels of instrumental support. A further study examining the perceived parental burden and service use for child and adolescent psychiatric disorders [9], found that 94% of caregivers reported at least one burden at some point during the 3 years of the study. It is therefore important to recognize the role of the parent for entry into a service pathway for a child with ADHD and how they can influence this. For adults with ADHD, there may be a similar role of the parent (if they are still living at home) or a partner, but no studies exist that evaluate the role of the parents or partners in determining if an adult with ADHD will seek help.

Costs of attention deficit hyperactivity disorder

The element of cost has been slowly appearing in the literature. It is discussed either as costs of providing a service (which appears to be mostly the interest of state-run health care systems) or societal costs from the condition (which is mostly the interest of humanist academics). The few studies that exist address all populations (children, adolescents, and adults) and come from the US and Europe [17,18], including the NICE Guidelines in the UK [19].

In trying to put a monetary value on ADHD in adults, the first study [20] made extrapolations of nongeneralizable data to calculate costs, so the final figures are not considered valid and are now obsolete. Of more interest is that the costs of the medicines for treatment of ADHD were reported to be approximately 7% of costs if "all other health care costs" and "work loss cost of adults with ADHD and adult family members" were added [20]. This would suggest that pharmacological treatment of adults with ADHD is cost-effective.

A comparison of costs between a generic medical service for chronic diseases and a service for adults with ADHD concluded that the service provision for ADHD poses an economic burden that is less than that of depression or diabetes, but greater than that of a seasonal allergy [21]; however, it is unclear how generalizable this conclusion is.

The topic of cost was taken up by European groups as well [22,23] and the difficulties of this undertaking were reported from the NICE perspective [24]. The first two studies identified that the ADHD during childhood results in significantly higher use of health care services and adversely affects academic achievement and parental productivity [23]. They also reported that there were higher mental health care costs for the mothers of ADHD patients [22]. These studies, although useful, only described what is observed by every clinician with experience of ADHD, and did not advance the literature by profiling specific sub-groups in enough detail so that interventions could be better targeted. For example, they did not evaluate if the parents had a specific mental health problem.

The literature studying the effects of ADHD in terms of employment costs is still in its infancy and reports significantly higher annual health benefit costs, absence days, and turnover for employees with ADHD, compared to employees without ADHD [25–30].

Trends in service delivery

A thorough study of the types of services provided to children identified as having ADHD was completed in the National Ambulatory Medical Care Survey in 1989, over a 7-year period [31]. This US study examined medication management, diagnostic services, mental health counseling, other counseling (ie, health-related advice), psychotherapy, and follow-up visits. What was recognized was that patterns of services for children with ADHD were changing with a marked increase in the numbers being assessed and treated for ADHD.

The identification of changes in service delivery is a consistent finding in the management of ADHD in both child and adult populations in many countries. The US study reported a doubling in the rate of diagnosing ADHD with the percentage of visits to physicians where ADHD was identified increasing from 0.74% in 1989 to 1.9% in 1996 [31]. This trend in prescribing and diagnosis has yet to be reversed and is most likely to be explained by the increased recognition of the disorder and the availability of effective treatments [31].

Local experiences and reports

In the UK, the increase in prescribing for ADHD has been documented using general practice prescription records. McCarthy and colleagues [32] investigated ADHD prescriptions in 15- to 22-year-olds and found an average 6.23-fold increase in the rates of prescribing between 1999 and 2006; this upward trend in prescription rates has continued since then [33]. Overall, the prescribing prevalence decreased markedly with age. In 2006, the prescribing rates in males dropped from 1.3% in 15-year olds to 0.06% in 21-year olds. Survival analysis showed that the rate of treatment cessation largely exceeded the estimated rate of persistence of ADHD [33]. The most notable reduction in treatment occurred between 16 and 17 years of age (Figure 11.1).

The same study also found that 18% of patients restarted treatment if they had stopped treatment after the age of 15 years [33]. Interviews

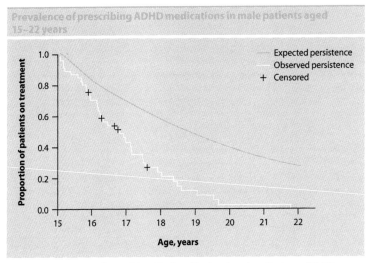

Figure 11.1 Prevalence of prescribing ADHD medications in male patients aged 15–22 years.
Reproduced with permission from McCarthy et al [32].

with a subset of young people found that although some found they could cope without medication, others felt the need to restart medication to gain control of ADHD symptoms. However, some of the patients interviewed reported difficulties re-engaging with services because of the lack of services to adults with ADHD. The difficulties experienced by adult patients with ADHD were recently documented in a qualitative study [34] from the same group (Figure 11.2) and in a further study from Adamou (Figure 11.3) [35]. Further quantitative research is clearly warranted of the basis of these qualitative findings to evaluate the true extent of unmet needs among adults with ADHD.

Pathways of care: a value-based approach

Currently, service delivery for adults with ADHD in the UK and across most of Europe, is often focused on the transition between child and

Adult attention deficit hyperactivity disorder patient experiences of impairments, service provision, and clinical management in England

- Patients diagnosed with ADHD reported that securing a definitive diagnosis was an 'uphill struggle,' often due to skeptical and negative attitudes toward ADHD health care professionals.
- ADHD-related impairment had an overwhelmingly chaotic impact on every aspect of patients' lives with which many patients felt ill equipped to cope, particularly among those who were not diagnosed until late adolescence or adulthood.
- A persistent sense of failure and missed potential from living with the impact of ADHD impairment had led to an accumulated psychosocial burden, particularly among those diagnosed from adolescence onward. In contrast, positive adjustment was facilitated by a younger age at diagnosis.
- Although pharmacological treatment was perceived as necessary in alleviating impairment, many felt strongly that medication by itself was inadequate. Additional support in the form of psychological therapies or psychoeducation was strongly desired, particularly amongst those diagnosed in adulthood. However, few patients had access to nonpharmacological treatment.
- In some, medication use was often inadequately monitored with little or no follow-up by health care professionals, leading to poor adherence and a sense of abandonment from the health care system. Participants also reported medication nonadherence and longer periods of medication cessation.

Conclusion: The findings suggest that the unmet needs of adults with ADHD are substantial and that there is a wide gap between stated policy and current practice in England. Greater awareness of ADHD in adults amongst health care professionals is needed to reduce or eliminate avoidable delays in diagnosis and to ensure that appropriate support for treatment management is provided. The results also suggest the need for augmenting existing pharmacological treatments with better psychological and educational support.

Figure 11.2 **Adult attention deficit hyperactivity disorder patient experiences of impairments, service provision, and clinical management in England.** Adapted from Matheson [34].

Effects of attention deficit hyperactivity disorder in adults: a grounded theory approach

Utilizing a grounded theory approach, seven themes emerged that represented health-related quality of life (HRQoL):

- Lack of a supportive network
- Labeling and attitudes from others
- Barriers placed on interpersonal relationships
- Psychological responses to ADHD
- Loss of opportunity to fulfill educational and occupational roles
- Therapeutic interventions
- Attitudes to medication

Conclusion: Although ADHD has been viewed mainly as a disorder of childhood, its impact on HRQoL of adults is significant. An ADHD service should expect that the needs of adults with ADHD will not be limited to pharmacological interventions but rather the facility should exist to offer interventions in a number of other domains

Figure 11.3 Effects of attention deficit hyperactivity disorder in adults: a grounded theory approach. ADHD, attention deficit hyperactivity disorder. Adapted from Adamou et al [35].

adolescent mental health services or pediatrics to adult mental health services. However, it is the experience of many new clinics that there is an even greater demand for assessment from those that were not diagnosed during childhood. This should come as no surprise, since we know that very few children were diagnosed before 1994 (in the UK and much of Europe) and numbers being treated in childhood continues to rise. It is to be expected that as child and adolescent services develop further and more children with ADHD are identified and offered treatment, the proportion of previously undiagnosed cases seeking assessments for ADHD as adults will reduce.

In terms of transitional care, when the frequency and content of transitional protocols was studied in the UK [6], disruption in continuity of care was identified [5], and this is considered to be a common problem across Europe [36]. This is consistent with the experience of UK community pediatricians who report that there have not been many places that their patients can go when they reach adulthood [37].

NICE recommendations

The right objective for health care is to increase value for patients, which is the quality of patient outcomes relative to the monies expended [38]. A safe approach to ensure that these quality outcomes are delivered is by having a service that is able to administer the clinical management recommendations from the NICE Guideline CG72 for ADHD across the lifespan [19]. This guideline includes diagnosis and treatment of ADHD in adults and provides an evidence-based review and recommendations for establishing an effective clinical care pathway and provision of services. It establishes the standards necessary for both transitional arrangements and first-time assessments for ADHD in adults and has led to a rapid increase in the number of local assessment teams; as yet, no formal evaluation has documented the expected improvements in clinical services. The following are key recommendations that guide the development of services:

- refer adults with ADHD symptoms of moderate or severe impairment to a mental health specialist in the diagnosis and treatment of ADHD;
- refer adults who were treated for ADHD in childhood and have symptoms suggestive of continuing ADHD to a mental health specialist in the diagnosis and treatment of ADHD;
- drug treatment should be the first-line treatment unless the person prefers psychological treatment;
- drug treatment for adults with ADHD should always form part of a comprehensive treatment program that addresses psychological, behavioral, and educational or occupational needs.

Service structure and determinants of service provision

There is little information to provide guidance on the best approach to establishing clinical services for adults with ADHD. There is a clear need for consistency and continuity of services, and to ensure that all aspects of the clinical care pathway are adequately catered for. In the UK there are relatively few dedicated services for adult ADHD patients or for adolescents reaching the age of 18; however, both the use of general and specialized adult mental health services has been successful in some cases. The NICE guidelines recognize that local arrangements for the delivery of mental health care will differ and establishing adequate services for ADHD in adults will require a detailed local assessment to ensure that all the required services are in place [19]. In general, three main approaches have been adopted in the UK and across Europe: specialist services, community mental health teams, and the consultative model.

Specialist service

One model for the delivery of services is the development of specialist services, working alongside primary care and based within Mental Health Trusts. Specialist services have the benefit of ensuring adequately trained staff with a particular interest in the management of ADHD. Furthermore, they may develop particular skills in delivering a broader range of support through psychoeducation, occupational therapy, psychological treatments and longer term support for adults with ADHD. In some parts of Europe it has been possible to develop lifespan services for ADHD, with continuity of care and professional expertise for ADHD at all ages. However, this does not match the service models of most regions. The establishment of local specialist services requires significant upfront investment, has a time lag until it is able to be productive, and its outcomes have yet to be fully evaluated.

Community Mental Health Teams standard model

Within the UK, community Mental Health Teams (CMHT) already have multidisciplinary teams (MDT) treating people with complex mental health problems. Although the boundaries for CMHT seem to be ever-changing, there is no reason why local expertise should not develop to include treatment of adults with ADHD as part of the standard service provision. Willingness to proceed along this route has been very weak in many regions, and it usually falls upon 'local champions' to take initiative, sometimes without support to deliver some care through their MDT.

Consultative model

Existing local professionals with expertise in ADHD are used to providing advice to CMHT so they can better manage their adult patients with ADHD. This model has evolved out of the 'local champions' trading their CMHT work for more specialist work for adults with ADHD. Although useful, this model can be expensive and also the treatment delivered will be at 'arms length' from the person with expertise.

Essential requirements

To be able to provide a patient-centric holistic diagnostic and treatment plan for an adult with ADHD, the service should be underpinned by the following:

- *Staffing:* professionals from many disciplines with appropriate training are able to offer a comprehensive assessment of medical, psychological and social needs including a risk assessment;
- *Treatments:* pharmacological, psychological, nursing, occupational, and social treatment should be available, although the specialist pathways for these have yet to be fully developed for adults with ADHD.
- *Links to other services:* links to other services are essential for the management of adults with ADHD. These include the following: general practitioners, substance misuse services, probation services, police service, prison service, educational institutions, employers forums, and support networks.

Referral sources

The following groups are expected to be referred to services for ADHD in adults (Figure 11.4):

- individuals with a previous history of childhood ADHD referred from pediatric services, Child and Adolescent Mental Health Services (CAMHS), or primary care;
- individuals with a previous history of treatment for childhood ADHD, who are no longer being monitored or treated;
- individuals who were not diagnosed with ADHD in childhood and where ADHD is recognized for the first time in adulthood.

The NICE guideline states that adults presenting with symptoms of ADHD in primary care who have not had a childhood diagnosis should be referred for assessment by adult psychiatric services trained in the diagnosis and treatment of ADHD, where there is evidence of typical manifestations of ADHD that:

- began during childhood and have persisted throughout life;
- are not better explained by other psychiatric diagnoses;
- have resulted in, or are associated with, moderate or severe psychological, social and/or occupational impairment [19].

Service group	Basic requirement
Stable and in-treatment for ADHD	• Prescriptions and health checks from primary care providers • Drug and/or psychological treatment monitoring from an ADHD specialist
Unstable or showing residual impairments; require review of medication and/or psychological treatments	• Access to adult mental health services for further assessment and treatment
Children/adolescents that have dropped out of treatment and now seeking further assessment in adulthood	• Access to adult mental health services for assessment and treatment
Adults with suspected ADHD (not previously diagnosed)	• Access to adult mental health services to assess for ADHD for the first time in adulthood

Figure 11.4 Attention deficit hyperactivity disorder service groups and their basic requirements. ADHD, attention deficit hyperactivity disorder.

Referral of young people with ADHD receiving treatment from CAMHS or pediatric services should be re-assessed at school-leaving age to establish whether there is a need for continued treatment and referral to adult services. If the young person does require further treatment, a formal meeting involving CAMHS and/or pediatrics and the adult psychiatric services is recommended. In order to ease the transition process, the Care Programme Approach may be adopted and, where possible, the young person should be involved in the planning of their ADHD management strategy.

Clinical care pathway

Based on these recommendations, a care pathway should be available for all those with suspected ADHD, or for those transitioning from child and adolescent to adult mental health services, with a previous diagnosis of ADHD (Figure 11.5).

Local arrangements need to be established for diagnostic assessment and the clinical management of all adults with ADHD. The basic services required to facilitate the clinical care pathway include:

• *Transition service:* arrangements for transition from child and adolescent to adult mental health services.
• *Diagnostic service*: first time diagnosis of adults with ADHD and those that 'fall out of treatment' and require a new assessment.

- *Drug monitoring service:* arrangements need to be in place for drug monitoring. This may be done by a specialist of generic adult mental health services, by appropriately trained psychiatrist or nurse practitioners, and by specialists working within primary care.
- *Psychological assessment and treatments:* psychological treatments are an essential component of clinical managements of ADHD in adults. Drug treatment should always be completed within the context of a comprehensive evaluation and provision for the psychosocial needs of patients.

Service requirements for patients with attention deficit hyperactivity disorder	
Step in clinical care pathway	**Service requirements**
A. Recognition of ADHD	Recognition of ADHD by primary or secondary care services. Clinicians need sufficient training to be able to recognize potential cases of ADHD
B. Screening for ADHD	Screening tools can be used to screen for ADHD (ASRS and/or current and childhood DSM-IV symptoms checklists)
C. Referral for diagnostic assessment	Adult patients with suspected ADHD should be referred to a specialist for diagnostic assessment. Referral information should include reasons for suspecting ADHD, outline of background developmental/psychiatric history and medical health check (cardiovascular function, pulse, blood pressure)
D. Clinical assessment	Diagnostic assessment and recommendations for treatment from appropriately trained specialist in adult ADHD
E. Prescribing medication	Prescribing of medication usually completed by primary care with shared care protocol in place
F. Monitoring drug treatments	Monitoring type and dose and continued need for medication by appropriately trained specialist
G. Psychological treatments	Provision of psychoeducation through group psychoeducation programs or as part of monitoring and support from specialist services. Treatment in the form of CBT, counseling and long-term support using approaches targeted at the specific psychological impairments experienced by adults with ADHD
H. Monitoring of psychological needs	Monitoring and provision of psychological support during routine monitoring and follow-up by primary care and specialist service

Figure 11.5 Service requirements for patients with attention deficit hyperactivity disorder. ADHD, attention deficit hyperactivity disorder. ASRS, Adult ADHD Self-Report Scale; CBT, cognitive behavioral therapy; DSM, *Diagnostic and Statistical Manual of Mental Disorders*. Adapted from Adamon [35].

Summary

The NICE Guideline CG72 [19] provides a good basic guide to what is required to be an effective treatment service for adults with ADHD. How this is delivered in the health care system is a matter that can be determined based on local circumstances or expertise. However, a more thorough understanding of referrers' needs, referral determinants, specialist multi-professional pathways, and patient recovery requirements will better allow us to design the appropriate service model for the future. The most immediate requirements are to ensure that services are provided for all steps in the clinical care pathway, to ensure that ADHD is recognized when it presents in adults, and that ADHD is properly diagnosed and treated.

References

1 Goldberg D, Huxley P. *Mental Illness in the Community: The Pathway to Psychiatric Care.* London: Tavistock; 1980.
2 Sayal K, Taylor E, Beecham J, Byrne P. Pathways to care in children at risk of attention-deficit hyperactivity disorder. *Br J of Psychiatry.* 2002;181:43-48.
3 Tettenborn M, Prasad S, Poole L, et al. The provision and nature of ADHD services for children/ adolescents in the UK: results from a nationwide survey. *Clin Child Psychol Psychiatry.* 2008;13:287-304.
4 Verity R, Coates J. Service innovation: transitional attention-deficit hyperactivity disorder clinic. *Psychiatr Bull.* 2007;31:99-100.
5 Singh SP. Transition of care from child to adult mental health services: the great divide. *Curr Opin Psychiatry.* 2009;22:386-390.
6 Singh SP, Paul M, Ford T, Kramer T, Weaver T. Transitions of care from Child and Adolescent Mental Health Services to Adult Mental Health Services (TRACK Study): a study of protocols in Greater London. *BMC Health Serv Res.* 2008;8:135.
7 Sayal K, Ford T, Goodman R. Trends in recognition of and service use for attention-deficit hyperactivity disorder in britain, 1999-2004. *Psychiatr Serv.* 2010;61:803-810.
8 Hoagwood K, Kelleher KJ, Feil M, Comer DM. Treatment services for children with ADHD: a national perspective. *J Am Acad Child Adolesc Psychiatry.* 2000;39:198-206.
9 Angold A, Erkanli A, Egger HL, Costello EJ. Stimulant treatment for children: a community perspective. *J Am Acad Child Adolesc Psychiatry.* 2000;39:975-894.
10 Wasserman RC, Kelleher KJ, Bocian A. Identification of attentional and hyperactivity problems in primary care: a report from pediatric research in office settings and the ambulatory sentinel practice network. *Pediatrics.* 1999;103:E38.
11 Zito JM, Safer DJ, dosReis S, Magder LS, Riddle MA. Methylphenidate patterns among Medicaid youths. *Psychopharmacol Bull.* 1997;33:143-147.
12 Gardner W, Kelleher KJ, Wasserman R, et al. Primary care treatment of pediatric psychosocial problems: A study from pediatric research in office settings and ambulatory sentinel practice network. *Pediatrics.* 2000;106:E44.
13 Nøvik TS, Hervas A, Ralston SJ, et al; for the ADORE Study Group. Influence of gender on attention-deficit/hyperactivity disorder in Europe-ADORE. *Eur Child Adolesc Psychiatry.* 2006;15:115-124.

14 Bussing R, Zima BT, Belin TR. Differential access to care for children with ADHD in special education programs. *Psychiatr Serv*. 1998;49:1226-1229.

15 Zito JM, Safer DJ, dosReis S, Riddle MA. Racial disparity in psychotropic medications prescribed for youths with Medicaid insurance in Maryland. *J Am Acad Child Adolesc Psychiatry*. 1998;37:179-184.

16 Bussing R, Zima BT, Gary FA, et al. Social networks, caregiver strain, and utilization of mental health services among elementary school students at high risk for ADHD. *J Am Acad Child Adolesc Psychiatry*. 2003;42:842-850.

17 Taylor E, Döpfner M, Sergeant J, et al. European clinical guidelines for hyperkinetic disorder - first upgrade. *Eur Child Adolesc Psychiatry*. 2004;13:17-30.

18 Taylor E, Sergeant J, Döpfner M, et al. Clinical guidelines for hyperkinetic disorder. European Society for Child and Adolescent Psychiatry. *Eur Child Adolesc Psychiatry*. 1998;7:184-200.

19 National Institute for Health and Clinical Excellence (NICE). NICE Guideline CG72: *Attention Deficit Hyperactivity Disorder: Diagnosis and Management of ADHD in Children, Young People and Adults*. NICE Website. www.nice.org.uk/CG72. Accessed August 24, 2012.

20 Birnbaum HG, Kessler RC, Lowe SW, et al. Costs of attention deficit-hyperactivity disorder (ADHD) in the US: excess costs of persons with ADHD and their family members in 2000. *Curr Med Res Opin*. 2005;21:195-206.

21 Hinnenthal JA, Perwien AR, Sterling KL. A comparison of service use and costs among adults with ADHD and adults with other chronic diseases. *Psychiatr Serv*. 2005;56:1593-1599.

22 Hakkaart-van Roijen L, Zwirs BW, Bouwmans C, et al. Societal costs and quality of life of children suffering from attention deficient hyperactivity disorder (ADHD*). Eur Child Adolesc Psychiatry*. 2007;16:316-326.

23 De Ridder A, De Graeve D. Healthcare use, social burden, and costs of children with and without ADHD in Flanders, Belgium. *Clin Drug Investig*. 2006;26:75-90.

24 Griffin SC, Weatherly HL, Richardson GA, Drummond MF. Methodological issues in undertaking independent cost-effectiveness analysis for NICE: the case of therapies for ADHD. *Eur J Health Econ*. 2008;9:137-145.

25 Kleinman NL, Durkin M, Melkonian A, Markosyan K. Incremental employee health benefit costs, absence days, and turnover among employees with ADHD and among employees with children with ADHD. *J Occup Environ Med*. 2009;51:1247-1255.

26 Kessler RC, Lane M, Stang PE, Van Brunt DL. The prevalence and workplace costs of adult attention deficit hyperactivity disorder in a large manufacturing firm. *Psychol Med*. 2009;39:137-147.

27 Halmoy A, Fasmer OB, Gillberg C, Haavik J. Occupational outcome in adult ADHD: impact of symptom profile, comorbid psychiatric problems, and treatment: a cross-sectional study of 414 clinically diagnosed adult ADHD patients. *J Atten Disord*. 2009;13:175-187.

28 de Graaf R, Kessler RC, Fayyad J, et al. The prevalence and effects of adult attention-deficit/hyperactivity disorder (ADHD) on the performance of workers: results from the WHO World Mental Health Survey Initiative. *Occup Environ Med*. 2008;65:835-842.

29 Kessler RC, Adler L, Ames M, et al. The prevalence and effects of adult attention deficit/hyperactivity disorder on work performance in a nationally representative sample of workers. *J Occup Environ Med*. 2005;47:565-572.

30 Barkley RA, Murphy KR. Impairment in occupational functioning and adult ADHD: the predictive utility of executive function (EF) ratings versus EF tests. *Arch Clin Neuropsychol*. 2010;25:157-173.

31 Kewley GD, Orford E. Attention deficit hyperactivity disorder is underdiagnosed and undertreated in Britain: Diagnosis needs tightening. *BMJ*. 1998;316:1594-1596.

32 McCarthy S, Asherson P, Coghill D, et al. Attention-deficit hyperactivity disorder: treatment discontinuation in adolescents and young adults. *Br J Psychiatry*. 2009;194:273-277.

33 Wong IC, Asherson P, Bilbow A, et al. Cessation of attention deficit hyperactivity disorder drugs in the young (CADDY)-a pharmacoepidemiological and qualitative study. *Health Technol Assess*. 2009;13:1-120.

34 Matheson L, Asherson P, Wong I, et al. P-876 – Adult ADHD patients' experiences of impairment, accessing services and treatment management - a qualitative study in England. *Eur Psychiatry.* 2012;27:1.

35 Adamou M. *Effects and Determinants of Service Provision for Adults with ADHD.* PhD Thesis. University of Kent; 2011.

36 Kooij SJ, Bejerot S, Blackwell A, et al. European consensus statement on diagnosis and treatment of adult ADHD: The European Network Adult ADHD. *BMC Psychiatry.* 2010;10:67.

37 Marcer H, Finlay F, Baverstock A. ADHD and transition to adult services-the experience of community paediatricians. *Child Care Health Dev.* 2008;34:564-566.

38 Report of the conference on the use of stimulant drugs in the treatment of behaviorally disturbed young school children. *Psychopharmacol Bull.* 1971;7:23-29.

Appendix A

UKAAN, *Handbook for Attention Deficit Hyperactivity Disorder in Adults*, DOI: 10.1007/978-1-908517-79-1, © Springer Healthcare 2013

Adult ADHD Self-Report Scale © (ASRS-v1.1) Symptom Checklist Instructions

The questions on the back page are designed to stimulate dialogue between you and your patients and to help confirm if they may be suffering from the symptoms of attention-deficit/hyperactivity disorder (ADHD)

Description: The symptom checklist is an instrument consisting of the 18 DSM-IV-TR criteria. Six of the 18 questions were found to be the most predictive of symptoms consistent with ADHD. These six questions are the basis for the ASRS v1.1 Screener and are also Part A of the Symptom Checklist. Part B of the Symptom Checklist contains the remaining 12 questions

Instructions

Symptoms

1. Ask the patient to complete both Part A and Part B of the symptom checklist by marking an X in the box that most closely represents the frequency of occurrence of each of the symptoms
2. Score Part A. If four or more marks appear in the darkly shaded boxes within Part A, then the patient has symptoms highly consistent with ADHD in adults and further investigation is warranted
3. The frequency scores on Part B provide additional cues and can serve as further probes into the patient's symptoms. Pay particular attention to marks appearing in the dark shaded boxes. The frequency-based response is more sensitive with certain questions. No total score or diagnostic likelihood is utilized for the twelve questions. It has been found that the six questions in Part A are the most predictive of the disorder and are best for use as a screening instrument

Impairments

1. Review the entire symptom checklist with your patients and evaluate the level of impairment associated with the symptom
2. Consider work/school, social, and family settings
3. Symptom frequency is often associated with symptom severity, therefore the symptom checklist may also aid in the assessment of impairments. If your patients have frequent symptoms, you may want to ask them to describe how these problems have affected the ability to work, take care of things at home, or get along with other people such as their spouse/significant other

History

1. Assess the presence of these symptoms or similar symptoms in childhood. Adults who have ADHD need not have been formally diagnosed in childhood. In evaluating a patient's history, look for evidence of early-appearing and long-standing problems with attention or self-control. Some significant symptoms should have been present in childhood, but full symptomology is not necessary

Adult ADHD Self-Report Scale © (ASRS-v1.1) Symptom Checklist

Name:	Date:					
Please answer the questions below, rating yourself on each of the criteria shown using the scale on the right side of the page. As you answer each question, place an X in the box that best describes how you have felt and conducted yourself over the past 6 months. Please give this completed checklist to your health care professional to discuss during today's appointment		Never	Rarely	Sometimes	Often	Very often
1.	How often do you have trouble wrapping up the final details of a project, once the challenging parts have been done?					
2.	How often do you have difficulty getting things in order when you have to do?					
3.	How often do you have problems remembering appointments or obligations?					
4.	When you have a task that requires a lot of thought, how often do you avoid or delay getting started?					
5.	How often do you fidget or squirm with your hands or feet when you have to sit down for a long time?					
6.	How often do you feel overly active and compelled to do things, like you were driven by a motor?					
7.	How often do you make careless mistakes when you have to work on a boring or difficult project?					
8.	How often do you have difficulty keeping your attention when you are doing boring or repetitive work?					
9.	How often do you have difficulty concentrating on what people say to you, even when they are speaking to you directly?					
10.	How often do you misplace or have difficulty finding things at home or at work?					
11.	How often are you distracted by activity or noise around you?					
12.	How often do you leave your seat in meetings or other situations in which you are expected to remain seated?					
13.	How often do you feel restless or fidgety?					
14.	How often do you have difficulty unwinding and relaxing when you have time to yourself?					
15.	How often do you find yourself talking too much when you are in social situations?					
16.	When you're in a conversation, how often do you find yourself finishing the sentences of the people you are talking to, before they can finish them themselves?					
17.	How often do you have difficulty waiting your turn in situations when turn taking is required?					
18.	How often do you interrupt others when they are busy?					

Appendix B

UKAAN, *Handbook for Attention Deficit Hyperactivity Disorder in Adults*, DOI: 10.1007/978-1-908517-79-1,
© Springer Healthcare 2013

Weiss Functional Impairment Rating Scale – Self report

Name: Date: /   /   (D/M/Y)

Date of birth: /   /   (D/M/Y)   Sex: ☐ Male ☐ Female

Work: ☐ Full-time ☐ Part-time ☐ Other: School: ☐ Full-time ☐ Part-time

Instructions: Circle the number for the rating that best describes how your emotional or behavioural problems have affected each item in the last month.

	Never or not at all	Sometimes or somewhat	Often or much	Very often or very much	Not applicable
A. Family					
1. Having problems with family	0	1	2	3	☐
2. Having problems with spouse/partner	0	1	2	3	☐
3. Relying on others to do things for you	0	1	2	3	☐
4. Causing fighting in the family	0	1	2	3	☐
5. Making it hard for the family to have fun together	0	1	2	3	☐
6. Problems taking care of your family	0	1	2	3	☐
7. Problems balancing your needs against those of your family	0	1	2	3	☐
8. Problems losing control with family	0	1	2	3	☐
B. Work					
1. Problems performing required duties	0	1	2	3	☐
2. Problems with getting your work done efficiently	0	1	2	3	☐
3. Problems with your supervisor	0	1	2	3	☐
4. Problems keeping a job	0	1	2	3	☐
5. Getting fired from work	0	1	2	3	☐
6. Problems working in a team	0	1	2	3	☐
7. Problems with your attendance	0	1	2	3	☐
8. Problems with being late	0	1	2	3	☐
9. Problems taking on new tasks	0	1	2	3	☐
10. Problems working to your potential	0	1	2	3	☐
11. Poor performance evaluations	0	1	2	3	☐
C. School					
1. Problems taking notes	0	1	2	3	☐
2. Problems completing assignments	0	1	2	3	☐
3. Problems getting your work done efficiently	0	1	2	3	☐
4. Problems with teachers	0	1	2	3	☐

Weiss Functional Impairment Rating Scale – Self report (continued)

	Never or not at all	Sometimes or somewhat	Often or much	Very often or very much	Not applicable
C. School (continued)					
5. Problems with school administrators	0	1	2	3	☐
6. Problems meeting minimum requirements to stay in school	0	1	2	3	☐
7. Problems with attendance	0	1	2	3	☐
8. Problems with being late	0	1	2	3	☐
9. Problems working to your potential	0	1	2	3	☐
10. Problems with inconsistent grades	0	1	2	3	☐
D. Life skills					
1. Excessive or inappropriate use of internet, video games, or TV	0	1	2	3	☐
2. Problems keeping an acceptable appearance	0	1	2	3	☐
3. Problems getting ready to leave the house	0	1	2	3	☐
4. Problems getting to bed	0	1	2	3	☐
5. Problems with nutrition	0	1	2	3	☐
6. Problems with sex	0	1	2	3	☐
7. Problems with sleeping	0	1	2	3	☐
8. Getting hurt or injured	0	1	2	3	☐
9. Avoiding exercise	0	1	2	3	☐
10. Problems keeping regular appointments with doctor/dentist	0	1	2	3	☐
11. Problems keeping up with household chores	0	1	2	3	☐
12. Problems managing money	0	1	2	3	☐
E. Life-concept					
1. Feeling bad about yourself	0	1	2	3	☐
2. Feeling frustrated with yourself	0	1	2	3	☐
3. Feeling discouraged	0	1	2	3	☐
4. Not feeling happy with your life	0	1	2	3	☐
5. Feeling incompetent	0	1	2	3	☐
F. Social					
1. Getting into arguments	0	1	2	3	☐
2. Trouble cooperating	0	1	2	3	☐
3. Trouble getting along with people	0	1	2	3	☐
4. Problems having fun with other people	0	1	2	3	☐
5. Problems participating in hobbies	0	1	2	3	☐

Weiss Functional Impairment Rating Scale – Self report (continued)

	Never or not at all	Sometimes or somewhat	Often or much	Very often or very much	Not applicable
F. Social (continued)					
6. Problems making friends	0	1	2	3	☐
7. Problems keeping friends	0	1	2	3	☐
8. Saying inappropriate things	0	1	2	3	☐
9. Complaints from neighbours	0	1	2	3	☐
G. Risk					
1. Aggressive driving	0	1	2	3	☐
2. Doing other things while driving	0	1	2	3	☐
3. Road rage	0	1	2	3	☐
4. Breaking or damaging things	0	1	2	3	☐
5. Doing things that are illegal	0	1	2	3	☐
6. Being involved with the police	0	1	2	3	☐
7. Smoking cigarettes	0	1	2	3	☐
8. Smoking marijuana	0	1	2	3	☐
9. Drinking alcohol	0	1	2	3	☐
10. Taking "street" drugs	0	1	2	3	☐
11. Sex without protection (birth control, condoms)	0	1	2	3	☐
12. Sexually inappropriate behaviour	0	1	2	3	☐
13. Being physically aggressive	0	1	2	3	☐
14. Being verbally aggressive	0	1	2	3	☐

Do not write in this area

A. Family	
B. Work	
C. School	
D. Life skills	
E. Self-concept	
F. Social	
G. Risk	
Total	

Reprinted with permission from Canadian ADHD Resource Alliance. University of British Columbia; 2011.

Appendix C

UKAAN, *Handbook for Attention Deficit Hyperactivity Disorder in Adults*, DOI: 10.1007/978-1-908517-79-1, © Springer Healthcare 2013

Current Behavior Scale – Self report

Instructions: Please circle the number next to each item that best describes your behavior
DURING THE PAST 6 MONTHS

Items	Never or rarely	Sometimes	Often	Very often
1. Fail to give close attention to details or made careless mistakes in my work	0	1	2	3
2. Fidget with hands or feet or squirm in seat	0	1	2	3
3. Have difficulty sustaining my attention in tasks or fun activities	0	1	2	3
4. Leave my seat in situations in which sitting is expected	0	1	2	3
5. Don't listen when spoken to directly	0	1	2	3
6. Feel restless	0	1	2	3
7. Don't follow through on instructions and fail to finish work	0	1	2	3
8. Have difficulty engaging in leisure activities or doing fun things quietly	0	1	2	3
9. Have difficulty organizing tasks and activities	0	1	2	3
10. Feel "on the go" or "driven by a motor"	0	1	2	3
11. Avoid, dislike, or am reluctant to engage in work that requires sustained mental effort	0	1	2	3
12. Talk excessively	0	1	2	3
13. Lose things necessary for tasks or activities	0	1	2	3
14. Blurt out answers before questions have been completed	0	1	2	3
15. Easily distracted	0	1	2	3
16. Have difficulty awaiting turn	0	1	2	3
17. Forgetful in daily activities	0	1	2	3
18. Interrupt or intrude on others	0	1	2	3

If you indicated that you experienced any of the problems with attention, concentration, impulsiveness, or hyperactivity on the first page, please fill in the blank below indicating as precisely as you can recall at what age these problems began to occur for you:

I was approximately _____ years old

To what extent do the problems you may have circled on the previous page interfere with your ability to function in each of these areas of life activities?

Areas	Never or rarely	Sometimes	Often	Very often
1. In your home life with your immediate family	0	1	2	3
2. In your work or occupation	0	1	2	3
3. In your social interactions with others	0	1	2	3
4. In your activities or dealings in the community	0	1	2	3
5. In any educational activities	0	1	2	3
6. In your dating or marital relationship	0	1	2	3
7. In your management of money	0	1	2	3
8. In your driving of a motor vehicle	0	1	2	3
9. In your leisure or recreational activities	0	1	2	3
10. In your management of your daily responsibilities	0	1	2	3

Current Behavior Scale – Self report (continued)

Reproduced with permissions from Barkley R, Murphy KR. Attention-Deficit Hyperactivity Disorder Workbook. New York, NY: Guildford Press; 2005.

Appendix D

UKAAN, *Handbook for Attention Deficit Hyperactivity Disorder in Adults*, DOI: 10.1007/978-1-908517-79-1, © Springer Healthcare 2013

Childhood Behavior Scale – Self report

Instructions: Please circle the number next to each item that best describes your behaviour when you were a child. **PLEASE RATE YOUR BEHAVIOUR BETWEEN 7 and 12 YEARS OF AGE**

Items	Never or rarely	Sometimes	Often	Very often
1. Failed to give close attention to details or made careless mistakes in my work	0	1	2	3
2. Fidgeted with hands or feet or squirmed in seat	0	1	2	3
3. Had difficulty sustaining my attention in tasks or fun activities	0	1	2	3
4. Left my seat in classroom or other situations in which sitting was expected	0	1	2	3
5. Didn't listen when spoken to directly	0	1	2	3
6. Restless in the "squirmy" sense	0	1	2	3
7. Didn't follow through on instructions and failed to finish work	0	1	2	3
8. Had difficulty engaging in leisure activities or doing fun things quietly	0	1	2	3
9. Had difficulty organizing tasks and activities	0	1	2	3
10. Felt "on the go" or acted as if "driven by a motor"	0	1	2	3
11. Avoided, disliked, or was reluctant to engage in work that required sustained mental effort	0	1	2	3
12. Talked excessively	0	1	2	3
13. Lost things necessary for tasks or activities	0	1	2	3
14. Blurted out answers before questions had been completed	0	1	2	3
15. Easily distracted	0	1	2	3
16. Had difficulty awaiting turn	0	1	2	3
17. Forgetful in daily activities	0	1	2	3
18. Interrupted or intruded on others	0	1	2	3

To what extent did the problems you may have circled on the previous page interfere with your ability to function in each of these areas of life activities **when you were a child between 7 and 12 years of age?**

Areas				
1. In your home life with your immediate family	0	1	2	3
2. In your social interactions with other children	0	1	2	3
3. In your activities or dealings in the community	0	1	2	3
4. In school	0	1	2	3
5. In sports, clubs, or other organizations	0	1	2	3
6. In learning to take care of yourself	0	1	2	3
7. In your play, leisure or recreational activities	0	1	2	3
8. In your handling of your daily chores or other responsibilities	0	1	2	3

Reproduced with permissions from Barkley R, Murphy KR. Attention-Deficit Hyperactivity Disorder Workbook. New York, NY: Guildford Press; 2005.

Appendix E

UKAAN, *Handbook for Attention Deficit Hyperactivity Disorder in Adults*, DOI: 10.1007/978-1-908517-79-1,
© Springer Healthcare 2013

Childhood Behavior Scale – Parent report

Instructions: Please circle the number next to each item that best describes the behaviour of your son or daughter when he or she was a child. **PLEASE RATE BEHAVIOUR AT AGE SEVEN (7 years of age)**

Items	Never or rarely	Sometimes	Often	Very often
1. Failed to give close attention to details or made careless mistakes in work	0	1	2	3
2. Fidgeted with hands or feet or squirmed in seat	0	1	2	3
3. Had difficulty sustaining attention in tasks or fun activities	0	1	2	3
4. Left seat in classroom or other situations in which sitting was expected	0	1	2	3
5. Didn't listen when spoken to directly	0	1	2	3
6. Restless in the "squirmy" sense	0	1	2	3
7. Didn't follow through on instructions and failed to finish work	0	1	2	3
8. Had difficulty engaging in leisure activities or doing fun things quietly	0	1	2	3
9. Had difficulty organizing tasks and activities	0	1	2	3
10. Was "on the go all the time" or acted as if "driven by a motor"	0	1	2	3
11. Avoided, disliked, or was reluctant to engage in work that required sustained mental effort	0	1	2	3
12. Talked excessively	0	1	2	3
13. Lost things necessary for tasks or activities	0	1	2	3
14. Blurted out answers before questions had been completed	0	1	2	3
15. Easily distracted	0	1	2	3
16. Had difficulty awaiting turn	0	1	2	3
17. Forgetful in daily activities	0	1	2	3
18. Interrupted or intruded on others	0	1	2	3

To what extent did the problems you may have circled on the previous page interfere with their ability to function in each of these areas of life activities, **when she or he was a child between 7 and 12 years of age?**

Areas				
1. In his/her home life with immediate family	0	1	2	3
2. In his/her social interactions with other children	0	1	2	3
3. In his/her activities or dealings in the community	0	1	2	3
4. In school	0	1	2	3
5. In sports, clubs, or other organizations	0	1	2	3
6. In learning to take care of themselves	0	1	2	3
7. In his/her play, leisure or recreational activities	0	1	2	3
8. In his/her handling of daily chores or other responsibilities	0	1	2	3

Reproduced with permissions from Barkley R, Murphy KR. Attention-Deficit Hyperactivity Disorder Workbook. New York, NY: Guildford Press; 2005.

Appendix F

UKAAN, *Handbook for Attention Deficit Hyperactivity Disorder in Adults*, DOI: 10.1007/978-1-908517-79-1, © Springer Healthcare 2013

Current Behavior Scale – Partner report

Instructions: Please circle the number next to each item that best describes your partner's behaviour **DURING THE PAST 6 MONTHS**

Items	Never or rarely	Sometimes	Often	Very often
1. Fails to give close attention to details or make careless mistakes in work	0	1	2	3
2. Fidgets with hands or feet or squirm in seat	0	1	2	3
3. Has difficulty sustaining attention in tasks or fun activities	0	1	2	3
4. Leaves seat in situations in which sitting is expected	0	1	2	3
5. Appears not to listen when spoken to directly	0	1	2	3
6. Appears restless	0	1	2	3
7. Does not follow through on instructions and fails to finish work	0	1	2	3
8. Has difficulty engaging in leisure activities or doing fun things quietly	0	1	2	3
9. Has difficulty organizing tasks and activities	0	1	2	3
10. Appears to be "on the go all the time" or as if "driven by a motor"	0	1	2	3
11. Avoids, dislikes, or is reluctant to engage in work that requires sustained mental effort	0	1	2	3
12. Talk excessively	0	1	2	3
13. Loses things necessary for tasks or activities	0	1	2	3
14. Blurts out answers before questions have been completed	0	1	2	3
15. Easily distracted	0	1	2	3
16. Has difficulty awaiting turn	0	1	2	3
17. Forgetful in daily activities	0	1	2	3
18. Interrupts or intrude on others	0	1	2	3

To what extent do the problems you may have circled on the previous page interfere with your partner's ability to function in each of these areas of life activities?

Areas				
1. In his/her home life with immediate family	0	1	2	3
2. In his/her work or occupation	0	1	2	3
3. In his/her social interactions with others	0	1	2	3
4. In his/her activities or dealings in the community	0	1	2	3
5. In any educational activities	0	1	2	3
6. In your dating or marital relationship	0	1	2	3
7. In his/her management of money	0	1	2	3
8. In his/her ability to drive a motor vehicle	0	1	2	3
9. In his/her leisure or recreational activities	0	1	2	3
10. In his/her management of daily responsibilities	0	1	2	3

Reproduced with permissions from Barkley R, Murphy KR. Attention-Deficit Hyperactivity Disorder Workbook. New York, NY: Guildford Press; 2005.

Appendix G

UKAAN, *Handbook for Attention Deficit Hyperactivity Disorder in Adults*, DOI: 10.1007/978-1-908517-79-1,
© Springer Healthcare 2013

Diagnostic Interview for ADHD in adults (DIVA)

The Diagnostic Interview for ADHD in adults (DIVA) is a publication of the DIVA Foundation, The Hague, The Netherlands, August 2010. The original English translation by Vertaalbureau Boot was supported by Janssen-Cilag B.V. Backtranslation into Dutch by Sietske Helder. Revison by Dr JJS Kooij, DIVA Foundation and Prof. Philip Asherson, Institute of Psychiatry, London

This publication has been put together with care. However, over the course of time, parts of this publication might change. For that reason, no rights may be derived from this publication. For more information and future updates of the DIVA please visit www.divacenter.eu

Introduction

According to the DSM-IV, ascertaining the diagnosis of ADHD in adults involves determining the presence of ADHD symptoms during both childhood and adulthood

The main requirements for the diagnosis are that the onset of ADHD symptoms occurred during childhood and that this was followed by a lifelong persistence of the characteristic symptoms to the time of the current evaluation. The symptoms need to be associated with significant clinical or psychosocial impairments that affect the individual in two or more life situations [1]. Because ADHD in adults is a lifelong condition that starts in childhood, it is necessary to evaluate the symptoms, course and level of associated impairment in childhood, using a retrospective interview for childhood behaviours. Whenever possible the information should be gathered from the patient and supplemented by information from informants that knew the person as a child (usually parents or close relatives) [2]

The Diagnostic Interview for ADHD in Adults (DIVA)

The DIVA is based on the DSM-IV criteria and is the first structured Dutch interview for ADHD in adults. The DIVA has been developed by JJS Kooij and MH Francken and is the successor of the earlier Semi-Structured Interview for ADHD in adults [2–3]

In order to simplify the evaluation of each of the 18 symptom criteria for ADHD, in childhood and adulthood, the interview provides a list of concrete and realistic examples, for both current and retrospective (childhood) behaviour. The examples are based on the common descriptions provided by adult patients in clinical practice. Examples are also provided of the types of impairments that are commonly associated with the symptoms in five areas of everyday life: work and education; relationships and family life; social contacts; free time and hobbies; self-confidence and self-image

Whenever possible the DIVA should be completed with adults in the presence of a partner and/or family member, to enable retrospective and collateral information to be ascertained at the same time. The DIVA usually takes around one and a half hours to complete

The DIVA only asks about the core symptoms of ADHD required to make the DSM-IV diagnosis of ADHD, and does not ask about other co-occurring psychiatric symptoms, syndromes or disorders. However comorbidity is commonly seen in both children and adults with ADHD, in around 75% of cases. For this reason, it is important to complete a general psychiatric assessment to enquire about commonly co-occurring symptoms, syndromes and disorders. The most common mental health problems that accompany ADHD include anxiety, depression, bipolar disorder, substance abuse disorders and addiction, sleep problems and personality disorders, and all these should be investigated. This is needed to understand the full range of symptoms experienced by the individual with ADHD; and also for the differential diagnosis, to exclude other major psychiatric disorders as the primary cause of 'ADHD symptoms' in adults [2]

Instructions for performing the DIVA

The DIVA is divided into three parts that are each applied to both childhood and adulthood:
(1) The criteria for Attention Deficit (A1)
(2) The criteria for Hyperactivity-Impulsivity (A2)
(3) The Age of Onset and Impairment accounted for by ADHD symptoms

Start with the first set of *DSM-IV criteria for attention deficit* (A1), followed by the second set of criteria for *hyperactivity/impulsivity* (A2). Ask about each of the 18 criteria in turn. For each item take the following approach:

First ask about adulthood (symptoms present in the last 6-months or more) and then ask about the same symptom in childhood (symptoms between the ages of 5 to 12 years) [4–6]. Read each question fully and ask the person being interviewed whether they recognise this problem and to provide examples. Patients will often give the same examples as those provided in the DIVA, which can then be ticked off as present. If they do not recognise the symptoms or you are not sure if their response is specific to the item in question, then use the examples, asking about each example in turn. For a problem behaviour or symptom to be scored as present, the problem should occur more frequently or at a more severe level than is usual in an age and IQ matched peer group, or to be closely associated with impairments. Tick off each of the examples that are described by the patient. If alternative examples that fit the criteria are given, make a note of these under 'other.' To score an item as present it is not necessary to score all the examples as present, rather the aim is for the investigator to obtain a clear picture of the presence or absence of each criterion

For each criterion, ask whether the partner or family member agrees with this or can give further examples of problems that relate to each item. As a rule, the partner would report on adulthood and the family member (usually parent or older relative) on childhood. The clinician has to use clinical judgement in order to determine the most accurate answer. If the answers conflict with one another, the rule of thumb is that the patient is usually the best informant [7]

The information received from the partner and family is mainly intended to supplement the information obtained from the patient and to obtain an accurate account of both current and childhood behaviour; the informant information is particularly useful for childhood since many patients have difficulty recalling their own behaviour retrospectively. Many people have a good recall for behaviour from around the age of 10–12 years of age, but have difficulty for the pre-school years

For each criterion, the researcher should make a decision about the presence or absence in both stages of life, taking into account the information from all the parties involved. If collateral information cannot be obtained, the diagnosis should be based on the patient's recall alone. If school reports are available, these can help to give an idea of the symptoms that were noticed in the classroom during childhood and can be used to support the diagnosis. Symptoms are considered to be clinically relevant if they occurred to a more severe degree and/or more frequently than in the peer group or if they were impairing to the individual

Age of onset and impairment

The third section on *Age of Onset and Impairment* accounted for by the symptoms is an essential part of the diagnostic criteria. Find out whether the patient has always had the symptoms and, if so, whether any symptoms were present before 7 years of age. If the symptoms did not commence till later in life, record the age of onset. Then ask about the examples for the different situations in which impairment can occur, first in adulthood then in childhood. Place a tick next to the examples that the patient recognises and indicate whether the impairment is reported for two or more domains of functioning. For the disorder to be present, it should cause impairment in at least two situations, such as work and education; relationships and family life; social contacts; free time and hobbies; self-confidence and self-image, and be at least moderately impairing

Diagnostic Interview for ADHD in adults (DIVA) (continued)

Summary of symptoms

In the *Summary of Symptoms of Attention Deficit* (A) *and Hyperactivity-Impulsivity* (HI), indicate which of the 18 symptom criteria are present in both stages of life; and sum the number of criteria for inattention and hyperactivity/impulsivity separately

Finally, indicate on the Score Form whether six or more criteria are scored for each of the symptom domains of Attention Deficit (A) and Hyperactivity-Impulsivity (HI). For each domain, indicate whether there was evidence of a lifelong persistent course for the symptoms, whether the symptoms were associated with impairment, whether impairment occurred in at least two situations, and whether the symptoms might be better explained by another psychiatric disorder. Indicate the degree to which the collateral information, and if applicable school reports, support the diagnosis. Finally, conclude whether the diagnosis of ADHD can be made and which subtype (with DSM-IV code) applies

Explanation to be given beforehand to the patient

This interview will be used to ask about the presence of ADHD symptoms that you experienced during your childhood and adulthood. The questions are based on the official criteria for ADHD in the DSM-IV. For each question I will ask you whether you recognise the problem. To help you during the interview I will provide some examples of each symptom, that describe the way that children and adults often experience difficulties related to each of the symptoms of ADHD. First of all, you will be asked the questions, then your partner and family members (if present) will be asked the same questions. Your partner will most likely have known you only since adulthood and will be asked questions about the period of your life that he or she knew you for; your family will have a better idea of your behaviour during childhood. Both stages of your life need to be investigated in order to be able to establish the diagnosis of ADHD

References

1. American Psychiatric Association (APA). *Diagnostic and Statistical Manual of Mental Disorders, 4th edn, text revision.* Washington DC: APA; 2000.
2. Diagnostic Interview for ADHD in Adults 2.0 (DIVA 2.0). In: Kooij JJS. *Adult ADHD. Diagnostic Assessment and Treatment.* Amsterdam: Pearson Assessment and Information BV; 2010.
3. Kooij, JJS, Francken MH. Diagnostisch Interview Voor ADHD (DIVA) bij volwassenen [Dutch]. www.kenniscentrumadhdbijvolwassenen. Accessed August 24, 2012.
4. Applegate B, Lahey BB, Hart EL, et al. Validity of the age-of-onset criterion for ADHD: a report from the DSM-IV field trials. *J Am Acad Child Adolesc Psychiatry.* 1997;36:1211-1221.
5. Barkley RA, Biederman J. Toward a broader definition of the age-of-onset criterion for attention-deficit hyperactivity disorder. *J Am Acad Child Adolesc Psychiatry.* 1997;36:1204-1210.
6. Faraone SV, Biederman J, Spencer T, et al. Diagnosing adult attention deficit hyperactivity disorder: are late onset and subthreshold diagnoses valid? *Am J Psychiatry.* 2006;163:1720-1709.
7. Kooij JJS, Boonstra AM, Willemsen-Swinkels SHN, Bekker EM, Noord Id, Buitelaar JL. Reliability, validity, and utility of instruments for self-report and informant report regarding symptoms of attention-deficit/hyperactivity disorder (ADHD) in adult patients. *J Atten Disorders.* 2008;11:445-458.

Reprinted with permission from the Diagnostic and Statistical Manual of Mental Disorders, Text Revision, Fourth Edition (Copyright 2000). American Psychiatric Association

Diagnostic Interview for ADHD in adults (DIVA) (continued)

Name of the patient:

Sex: ☐ Male

Date of birth: /   /   ☐ Female   Date of interview: /   /

Name of researcher:

Part 1: Symptoms of attention-deficit (DSM-IV criterion A1)

Instructions: The symptoms in adulthood have to have been present for at least 6 months. The symptoms in childhood relate to the age of 5–12 years. For a symptom to be ascribed to ADHD, it should have a chronic trait-like course and should not be episodic

A1: Do you often fail to give close attention to detail, or do you make careless mistakes in your work or during other activities? And how was that during childhood?

Examples during adulthood:

☐ Makes careless mistakes

☐ Works slowly to avoid mistakes

☐ Does not read instructions carefully

☐ Difficulty working in a detailed way

☐ Too much time needed to complete detailed tasks

☐ Gets easily bogged down by details

☐ Works too quickly and therefore makes mistakes

☐ Other:

Symptom present: ☐ Yes ☐ No

Examples during childhood:

☐ Careless mistakes in schoolwork

☐ Mistakes made by not reading questions properly

☐ Leaves questions unanswered by not reading them properly

☐ Leaves the reverse side of a test unanswered

☐ Others comment about careless work

☐ Not checking the answers in homework

☐ Too much time needed to complete detailed tasks

☐ Other:

Symptom present: ☐ Yes ☐ No

A2: Do you often find it difficult to sustain your attention on tasks? And how was that during childhood?

Examples during adulthood:

☐ Not able to keep attention on tasks for long*

☐ Quickly distracted by own thoughts or associations

☐ Finds it difficult to watch a film through to the end, or to read a book*

☐ Quickly becomes bored with things*

☐ Asks questions about subjects that have already been discussed

☐ Other:

Unless the subject is found to be really interesting (eg, computer or hobby)

Symptom present: ☐ Yes   ☐ No

Examples during childhood:

☐ Difficulty keeping attention on schoolwork

☐ Difficulty keeping attention on play*

☐ Easily distracted

☐ Difficulty concentrating*

☐ Needing structure to avoid becoming distracted

☐ Quickly becoming bored of activities*

☐ Other:

Unless the subject is found to be really interesting (eg, computer or hobby)

Symptom present: ☐ Yes   ☐ No

A3: Does it often seem as though you are not listening when you are spoken to directly? And how was that during childhood?

Examples during adulthood:

☐ Dreamy or preoccupied

☐ Difficulty concentrating on a conversation

☐ Afterwards, not knowing what a conversation was about

☐ Often changing the subject of the conversation

☐ Others saying that your thoughts are somewhere else

☐ Other:

Symptom present: ☐ Yes   ☐ No

Examples during childhood:

☐ Not knowing what parents/teachers have said

☐ Dreamy or preoccupied

☐ Only listening during eye contact or when a voice is raised

☐ Often having to be addressed again

☐ Questions having to be repeated

☐ Other:

Symptom present: ☐ Yes   ☐ No

Diagnostic Interview for ADHD in adults (DIVA) (continued)

A4: Do you often fail to follow through on instructions and do you often fail to finish jobs or fail to meet obligations at work? And how was that during childhood (when doing schoolwork as opposed to when at work)?

Examples during adulthood:

☐ Does things that are muddled up together without completing them

☐ Difficulty completing tasks once the novelty has worn off

☐ Needing a time limit to complete tasks

☐ Difficulty completing administrative tasks

☐ Difficultly following instructions from a manual

☐ Other:

Symptom present: ☐ Yes   ☐ No

Examples during childhood:

☐ Difficulty following instructions

☐ Difficulty with instructions involving more than one step

☐ Not completing things

☐ Not completing homework or handing it in

☐ Needing a lot of structure in order to complete tasks

☐ Other:

Symptom present: ☐ Yes   ☐ No

A5: Do you often find it difficult to organise tasks and activities? And how was that during childhood?

Examples during adulthood:

☐ Difficultly with planning activities of daily life

☐ House and/or workplace are disorganised

☐ Planning too many tasks or nonefficient planning

☐ Regularly booking things to take place at the same time (double-booking)

☐ Arriving late

☐ Not able to use an agenda or diary consistently

☐ Inflexible because of the need to keep to schedules

☐ Poor sense of time

☐ Creating schedules but not using them

☐ Needing other people to structure things

☐ Other:

Symptom present: ☐ Yes   ☐ No

Examples during childhood:

☐ Difficultly being ready on time

☐ Messy room or desk

☐ Difficultly playing alone

☐ Difficulty planning tasks or homework

☐ Doing things in a muddled way

☐ Arriving late

☐ Poor sense of time

☐ Difficulty keeping himself/herself entertained

☐ Other:

Symptom present: ☐ Yes ☐ No

A6: Do you often avoid (or do you have an aversion to, or are you unwilling to do) tasks which require sustained mental effort? And how was that during childhood?

Examples during adulthood:

☐ Do the easiest or nicest things first of all

☐ Often postpone boring or difficult tasks

☐ Postpone tasks so that deadlines are missed

☐ Avoid monotonous work, such as administration

☐ Do not like reading due to mental effort

☐ Avoidance of tasks that require a lot of concentration

☐ Other:

Symptom present: ☐ Yes ☐ No

Examples during childhood:

☐ Avoidance of homework or has an aversion to this

☐ Reads few books or does not feel like reading due to mental effort

☐ Avoidance of tasks that require a lot of concentration

☐ Aversion to school subjects that require a lot of concentration

☐ Often postpones boring or difficult tasks

☐ Other:

Symptom present: ☐ Yes ☐ No

A7: Do you often lose things that are needed for tasks or activities? And how was that during childhood?

Examples during adulthood:

☐ Mislays wallet, keys, or agenda

☐ Often leaves things behind

☐ Loses papers for work

☐ Loses a lot of time searching for things

☐ Gets in a panic if other people move things around

Diagnostic Interview for ADHD in adults (DIVA) (continued)

☐ Stores things away in the wrong place

☐ Loses notes, lists, or telephone numbers

☐ Other:

Symptom present: ☐ Yes ☐ No

Examples during childhood:

☐ Loses diaries, pens, gym kit, or other items

☐ Mislays toys, clothing, or homework

☐ Spends a lot of time searching for things

☐ Gets in a panic if other people move things around

☐ Comments from parents and/or teacher about things being lost

☐ Other:

Symptom present: ☐ Yes ☐ No

A8: Are you often easily distracted by external stimuli? And how was that during childhood?

Examples during adulthood:

☐ Difficulty shutting off from external stimuli

☐ After being distracted, difficult to pick up the thread again

☐ Easily distracted by noises or events

☐ Easily distracted by the conversations of others

☐ Difficulty in filtering and/or selecting information

☐ Other:

Symptom present: ☐ Yes ☐ No

Examples during childhood:

☐ In the classroom, often looking outside

☐ Easily distracted by noises or events

☐ After being distracted, has difficultly picking up the thread again

☐ Other:

Symptom present: ☐ Yes ☐ No

A9: Are you often forgetful during daily activities? And how was that during childhood?

Examples during adulthood:

☐ Forgets appointments or other obligations

☐ Forgets keys, agenda, etc

☐ Needs frequent reminders for appointments

☐ Returning home to fetch forgotten things

☐ Rigid use of lists to make sure things aren't forgotten

☐ Forgets to keep or look at daily agenda

☐ Other:

Symptom present: ☐ Yes ☐ No

Examples during childhood:

☐ Forgets appointments or instructions

☐ Has to be frequently reminded of things

☐ Half-way through a task, forgetting what has to be done

☐ Forgets to take things to school

☐ Leaving things behind at school or at friends' houses

☐ Other:

Symptom present: ☐ Yes ☐ No

Supplement criterion A

Adulthood
Do you have more of these symptoms of attention deficit than other people, or do you experience these more frequently than other people of your age?

☐ Yes ☐ No

Childhood
Did you have more of these symptoms of attention deficit than other children of your age, or did you experience these more frequently than other children of your age?

☐ Yes ☐ No

Part 2: Symptoms of hyperactivity-impulsivity (DSM-IV criterion A2)

Instructions: the symptoms in adulthood have to have been present for at least 6 months. The symptoms in childhood relate to the age of 5–12 years. For a symptom to be ascribed to ADHD, it should have a chronic trait-like course and should not be episodic

H/I 1: Do you often move your hands or feet in a restless manner, or do you often fidget in your chair? And how was that during childhood?

Examples during adulthood:

☐ Difficulty sitting still

☐ Fidgets with the legs

☐ Tapping with a pen or playing with something

☐ Fiddling with hair or biting nails

☐ Able to control restlessness but feels stressed as a result

☐ Other:

Symptom present: ☐ Yes ☐ No

Examples during childhood:

☐ Parents often said "sit still" or similar

☐ Fidgets with the legs

☐ Tapping with a pen or playing with something

☐ Fiddling with hair or biting nails

☐ Unable to remain seated in a chair in a relaxed manner

☐ Able to control restlessness, but feels stressed as a result

☐ Other:

Symptom present: ☐ Yes ☐ No

H/I 2: Do you often stand up in situations where the expectation is that you should remain in your seat? And how was that during childhood?

Examples during adulthood:

☐ Avoids symposiums, lectures, church, etc

☐ Prefers to walk around rather than sit

☐ Never sits still for long, always moving around

☐ Stressed owing to the difficulty of sitting still

☐ Makes excuses in order to be able to walk around

☐ Other:

Symptom present: ☐ Yes ☐ No

Examples during childhood:

☐ Often stands up while eating or in the classroom

☐ Finds it very difficult to stay seated at school or during meals

☐ Being told to remain seated

☐ Making excuses in order to walk around

☐ Other:

Symptom present: ☐ Yes ☐ No

H/I 3: Do you often feel restless? And how was that during childhood?

Examples during adulthood:

☐ Feeling restless or agitated inside

☐ Constantly having the feeling that you have to be doing something

☐ Finding it hard to relax

☐ Other:

Symptom present: ☐ Yes ☐ No

Examples during childhood:

☐ Always running around

☐ Climbing on furniture, or jumping on the sofa

☐ Climbing in trees

☐ Feeling restless inside

☐ Other:

Symptom present: ☐ Yes ☐ No

H/I 4: Do you often find it difficult to engage in leisure activities quietly? And how was that during childhood?

Examples during adulthood:

☐ Talks during activities when this is not appropriate

☐ Becoming quickly too cocky in public

☐ Being loud in all kinds of situations

☐ Difficulty doing activities quietly

☐ Difficultly in speaking softly

☐ Other:

Symptom present: ☐ Yes ☐ No

Examples during childhood:

☐ Being loud-spoken during play or in the classroom

☐ Unable to watch TV or films quietly

☐ Asked to be quieter or calm down

☐ Becoming quickly too cocky in public

☐ Other:

Symptom present: ☐ Yes ☐ No

H/I 5: Are you often on the go or do you often act as if "driven by a motor"? And how was that during childhood?

Examples during adulthood:

☐ Always busy doing something

☐ Has too much energy, always on the move

☐ Stepping over own boundaries

☐ Finds it difficult to let things go, excessively driven

☐ Other:

Symptom present: ☐ Yes ☐ No

Examples during childhood:

☐ Constantly busy

☐ Excessively active at school and at home

☐ Has lots of energy

☐ Always on the go, excessively driven

☐ Other:

Symptom present: ☐ Yes ☐ No

H/I 6: Do you often talk excessively? And how was that during childhood?

Examples during adulthood:

☐ So busy talking that other people find it tiring

☐ Known to be an incessant talker

☐ Finds it difficult to stop talking

☐ Tendency to talk too much

☐ Not giving others room to interject during a conversation

☐ Needing a lot of words to say something

☐ Other:

Symptom present: ☐ Yes ☐ No

Examples during childhood:

☐ Known as a chatterbox

☐ Teachers and parents often ask you to be quiet

☐ Comments in school reports about talking too much

☐ Being punished for talking too much

☐ Keeping others from doing schoolwork by talking too much

☐ Not giving others room during a conversation

☐ Other:

Symptom present: ☐ Yes   ☐ No

H/I 7: Do you often give the answer before questions have been completed? And how was that during childhood?

Examples during adulthood:

☐ Being a blabbermouth, saying what you think

☐ Saying things without thinking first

☐ Giving people answers before they have finished speaking

☐ Completing other people's words

☐ Being tactless

☐ Other:

Symptom present: ☐ Yes   ☐ No

Examples during childhood:

☐ Being a blabbermouth, saying things without thinking first

☐ Wants to be the first to answer questions at school

☐ Blurts out an answer even if it is wrong

☐ Interrupts others before sentences are finished

☐ Coming across as being tactless

☐ Other:

Symptom present: ☐ Yes   ☐ No

H/I 8: Do you often find it difficult to await your turn? And how was that during childhood?

Examples during adulthood:

☐ Difficulty waiting in a queue, jumping the queue

☐ Difficulty in patiently waiting in the traffic/traffic jams

☐ Difficulty waiting your turn during conversations

☐ Being impatient

☐ Quickly starting relationships/jobs, or ending/leaving these because of impatience

☐ Other:

Examples during childhood:

☐ Difficultly waiting turn in group activities

☐ Difficultly waiting turn in the classroom

☐ Always being the first to talk or act

☐ Becomes quickly impatient

☐ Crosses the road without looking

☐ Other:

Symptom present: ☐ Yes ☐ No

H/I 9: Do you often interrupt the activities of others, or intrude on others? And how was that during childhood?

Examples during adulthood:

☐ Being quick to interfere with others

☐ Interrupts others

☐ Disturbes other people's activities without being asked

☐ Comments from others about interference

☐ Difficulty respecting the boundaries of others

☐ Having an opinion about everything and immediately expressing this

☐ Other:

Symptom present: ☐ Yes ☐ No

Examples during childhood:

☐ Impinges on the games of others

☐ Interrupts the conversations of others

☐ Reacts to everything

☐ Unable to wait

☐ Other:

Symptom present: ☐ Yes ☐ No

Supplement criterion A

Adulthood

Do you have more of these symptoms of hyperactivity/impulsivity than other people,   ☐ Yes
or do you experience these more frequently than other people?   ☐ No

Childhood

Did you have more of these symptoms of hyperactivity/impulsivity than other children of   ☐ Yes
your age, or did you experience these more frequently than other children of your age?   ☐ No

Part 3: Impairment on account of the symptoms (DSM-IV criteria B, C and D)

Criterion B

Have you always had these symptoms of attention deficit and/or hyperactivity/impulsivity?

☐ Yes (a number of symptoms were present prior to the 7th year of age)

☐ No

If no is answered above, starting as from _____ year of age

Criterion C

Adulthood

In which areas do you have / have you had problems with these symptoms?

Work/education

☐ Did not complete education/training needed for work

☐ Work below level of education

☐ Tire quickly of a workplace

☐ Pattern of many short-lasting jobs

☐ Difficulty with administrative work/planning

☐ Not achieving promotions

☐ Under-performing at work

☐ Left work following arguments or dismissal

☐ Sickness benefits/disability benefit as a result of symptoms

☐ Limited impairment through compensation of high IQ

☐ Limited impairment through compensation of external structure

☐ Other:

Relationship and/or family

☐ Tire quickly of relationships

☐ Impulsively commencing/ending relationships

☐ Unequal partner relationship owing to symptoms

☐ Relationship problems, lots of arguments, lack of intimacy

☐ Divorced owing to symptoms

☐ Problems with sexuality as a result of symptoms

☐ Problems with upbringing as a result of symptoms

☐ Difficulty with housekeeping and/or administration

☐ Financial problems or gambling

☐ Not daring to start a relationship

☐ Other:

Social contacts

☐ Tire quickly of social contacts

☐ Difficultly maintaining social contacts

☐ Conflicts as a result of communication problems

☐ Difficulty initiating social contacts

☐ Low self-assertiveness as a result of negative experiences

☐ Not being attentive (ie, forget to send a card/empathising/phoning, etc)

☐ Other:

Free time/hobby

☐ Unable to relax properly during free time

☐ Having to play lots of sports in order to relax

☐ Injuries as a result of excessive sport

☐ Unable to finish a book or watch a film all the way through

☐ Being continually busy and therefore becoming overtired

☐ Tire quickly of hobbies

☐ Accidents/loss of driving licence as a result of reckless driving behaviour

☐ Sensation seeking and/or taking too many risks

☐ Contact with the police/the courts

☐ Binge eating

☐ Other:

Self-confidence/self-image

☐ Uncertainty through negative comments of others

☐ Negative self-image due to experiences of failure

☐ Fear of failure in terms of starting new things

☐ Excessive intense reaction to criticism

☐ Perfectionism

☐ Distressed by the symptoms of ADHD

☐ Other:

Childhood and adolescence

In which areas do you have / have you had problems with these symptoms?

Education

☐ Lower educational level than expected based on IQ

☐ Staying back (repeating classes) as a result of concentration problems

☐ Education not completed/rejected from school

☐ Took much longer to complete education than usual

☐ Achieved education suited to IQ with a lot of effort

☐ Difficulty doing homework

☐ Followed special education on account of symptoms

☐ Comments from teachers about behaviour or concentration

☐ Limited impairment through compensation of high IQ

☐ Limited impairment through compensation of external structure

☐ Other:

Family

☐ Frequent arguments with brothers or sisters

☐ Frequent punishment or hiding

☐ Little contact with family on account of conflicts

☐ Required structure from parents for a longer period than would normally be the case

☐ Other:

Social contacts

☐ Difficultly maintaining social contacts

☐ Conflicts as a result of communication problems

☐ Difficultly entering into social contacts

☐ Low self-assertiveness as a result of negative experiences

☐ Few friends

☐ Being teased

☐ Shut out by, or not being allowed to do things with, a group

☐ Being a bully

☐ Other:

Free time/hobby

☐ Unable to relax properly during free time

☐ Having to play lots of sport to be able to relax

☐ Injuries as a result of excessive sport

☐ Unable to finish a book or watch a film all the way through

☐ Being continually busy and therefore becoming overtired

☐ Tired quickly of hobbies

☐ Sensation seeking and/or taking too many risks

☐ Contact with the police/courts

☐ Increased number of accidents

☐ Other:

Self-confidence/self-image

☐ Uncertainty through negative comments of others

☐ Negative self-image due to experiences of failure

☐ Fear of failure in terms of starting new things

☐ Excessive intense reaction to criticism

☐ Perfectionism

☐ Other:

Adulthood
Evidence of impairment in two or more areas?   ☐ Yes ☐ No

Childhood and adolescence
Evidence of impairment in two or more areas?   ☐ Yes ☐ No

End of the interview. Please continue with the summary

Potential details:

Summary of symptoms A and H/I

Indicate which criteria were scored in parts 1 and 2 and add up

Criterion DSM-IV TR	Symptom		Present during adulthood	Present during childhood
A1a	A1	Often fails to pay close attention to details, or makes careless mistakes in schoolwork, work or during other activities		
A1b	A2	Often has difficultly sustaining attention in tasks or play		
A1c	A3	Often does not seem to listen when spoken to directly		
A1d	A4	Often does not follow through on instructions and fails to finish schoolwork, chores, or duties in the workplace		
A1e	A5	Often has difficulty organizing tasks and activities		
A1f	A6	Often avoids, dislikes, or is reluctant to engage in tasks that require sustained mental effort (such as school of homework)		
A1g	A7	Often loses things necessary for tasks or activities		
A1h	A8	Often easily distracted by extraneous stimuli		
A1i	A9	Often forgetful in daily activities		
Total number of criteria attention deficit			/9	/9
A2a	H/I 1	Often fidgets with hands or feet or squirms in seat		
A2b	H/I 2	Often leaves seat in classroom or in other situations in which remaining seated is expected		
A2c	H/I 3	Often runs about or climbs excessively in situations in which it is inappropriate (in adolescents or adults this may be limited to subjective feelings of restlessness)		
A2d	H/I 4	Often has difficulty playing or engaging in leisure activities quietly		
A2e	H/I 5	Is often on the go or often acts as if 'driven by a motor'		
A2f	H/I 6	Often talks excessively		

Diagnostic Interview for ADHD in adults (DIVA) (continued)

Criterion DSM-IV TR	Symptom	Present during adulthood	Present during childhood
A2g	H/I 7 Often blurts out answers before questions have been completed		
A2h	H/I 8 Often has difficulty awaiting turn		
A2i	H/I 9 Often interrupts or intrudes on others		
Total number of criteria hyperactivity/impulsivity		/9	/9
Score form			
DSM-IV criterion A	**Childhood** Is the number of A characteristics ≥6? Is the number of H/I characteristics ≥6? **Adulthood*** Is the number of A characteristics ≥6? Is the number of H/I characteristics ≥6?	☐ Yes ☐ No ☐ Yes ☐ No ☐ Yes ☐ No ☐ Yes ☐ No	
DSM-IV criterion B	Are there signs of a lifelong pattern of symptoms and limitations?	☐ Yes ☐ No	
DSM-IV criterion C and D	The symptoms and the impairment are expressed in at least two domains of functioning Adulthood Childhood	 ☐ Yes ☐ No ☐ Yes ☐ No	
DSM-IV criterion E	The symptoms cannot be (better) explained by the presence of another psychiatric disorder	☐ No Yes, by: _____	
	Is the diagnosis supported by collateral information? Parent(s)/brother/sister/other, ie, _____ [†] Partner/good friend/other, ie, _____ [†] School reports 0 = none/little support 1 = some support 2 = clear support	 ☐ N/A ☐ 0 ☐ 1 ☐ 2 ☐ N/A ☐ 0 ☐ 1 ☐ 2 ☐ N/A ☐ 0 ☐ 1 ☐ 2 Explanation:	
	Diagnosis ADHD[‡]	☐ No Yes, subtype ☐ 314.01 Combined type ☐ 314.00 Predominantly inattentive type ☐ 314.01 Predominantly hyperactive-impulsive type	

*Research has indicated that at adult age, four or more characteristics of attention problems and/ or hyperactivity-impulsivity are sufficient for the diagnosis of ADHD to be made. Reprinted with permission from DIVA Foundation 2010. www.divacentre.eu

† Indicate from whom the collateral information was taken

‡ If the established sub-types differ in childhood and adulthood, the current adult sub-type prevails for the diagnosis

Appendix H

UKAAN, *Handbook for Attention Deficit Hyperactivity Disorder in Adults*, DOI: 10.1007/978-1-908517-79-1,
© Springer Healthcare 2013

Medical Assessment Tool for Adults with ADHD

Have you ever been told by a doctor that you have heart disease?

Do you ever get chest pain on exertion?

Have you ever passed out or fainted whilst exercising?

Has anyone in your family developed heart disease before the age of 60 years?

Has anyone in your family died of heart disease before the age of 60 years?

Do you know if you have high blood pressure or an increased cholesterol

Blood pressure/pulse - is it regular?

Healthy weight?

Physical examination including pulse, blood pressure and examination for heart murmurs

ECG, ECHO, and 24-hour blood pressure (if indicated)

Appendix I

UKAAN, *Handbook for Attention Deficit Hyperactivity Disorder in Adults*, DOI: 10.1007/978-1-908517-79-1,
© Springer Healthcare 2013

Service for adults with ADHD referral form - example

Patient name:	Date of birth: / /	(D/M/Y)

Address:

Contact phone number:

General practitioner information

Name: Phone number:

Address:

Professionals involved

CMHT locality (if applicable):

Responsible clinician:

CPA Care Co-ordinator (if applicable):

Other:

Survey

Is person in agreement with referral?	☐ Yes ☐ No

What are their expectations from our service?

Has a parent/carer been consulted about referral (if client under 18)?	☐ Yes ☐ No
Have referrals been made to other agencies/organisations?	☐ Yes ☐ No

If so which?

The following documentation must be included with this referral form unless available electronically (Please note that assessments will be delayed until this is supplied).

1. Clinical report*	☐ Yes ☐ No
2. CPA (if applicable, no more than 3 months old)	☐ Yes ☐ No
3. Risk assessment	☐ Yes ☐ No

Please see next page for details

Signature: Base:

(Please print name)

Telephone: Date: / / (D/M/Y)

Email address:

Service for adults with ADHD referral form - example (continued)

Clinical report

The clinical report should include the following information:

Current presentation including:
- current mental state
- motivation
- attitude to treatment
- daily routine
- activity levels
- engagement

Social support networks

Benefits and housing (if applicable)

Behavioral analysis and previous intervention programs

Level of functional ability

Employment/education status

Client's priorities, goals, and aspirations

Psychiatric history including:
- history of present circumstances
- family history
- personal history
- social history
- past psychiatric history
- forensic history (if relevant)
- medical history
- medication
- drug and alcohol history
- outcome of any interventions

Appendix J

UKAAN, *Handbook for Attention Deficit Hyperactivity Disorder in Adults*, DOI: 10.1007/978-1-908517-79-1, © Springer Healthcare 2013

Clinical Global Impression

1. Severity of illness

Considering your total clinical experience with this particular population, how mentally ill is the patient at this time?

0 = Not assessed
1 = Normal, not at all ill
2 = Borderline mentally ill
3 = Mildly ill
4 = Moderately ill
5 = Markedly ill
6 = Severely ill
7 = Among the most extremely ill patients

Global improvement: rate total improvement whether or not, in your judgement, it is due entirely to drug treatment

Compared to his condition at admission to the project, how much has he changed?

0 = Not assessed
1 = Very much improved
2 = Much improved
3 = Minimally improved
4 = No change
5 = Minimally worse
6 = Much worse
7 = Very much worse

Efficacy index: Rate this item on the basis of *drug effect only*.

Select the terms which best describe the degrees of therapeutic effect and side effects and record the number in the box where the two items intersect

EXAMPLE: Therapeutic effect is rated as 'Moderate' and side effects are judged 'Do not significantly interfere with patient's functioning'

		Side effects			
Therapeutic effect		**None**	**Do not interfere**	**Significantly interferes**	**Outweighs therapeutic effect**
Marked	Vast improvement. Complete or nearly complete remission of all symptoms	01	02	03	04
Moderate	Decided improvement. Partial remission of symptoms	05	06	07	08
Minimal	Slight improvement which doesn't alter status of care of patient	09	10	11	12
Unchanged or worse		13	14	15	16

Not assessed = 00

Reproduced from Guy W, editor. ECDEU Assessment Manual for Psychopharmacology. 1976. Rockville, MD, U.S. Department of Health, Education, and Welfare

Appendix K

UKAAN, *Handbook for Attention Deficit Hyperactivity Disorder in Adults*, DOI: 10.1007/978-1-908517-79-1,
© Springer Healthcare 2013

Attention deficit hyperactivity disorder clinical assessment summary

Name: Date of birth: /   /   (D/M/Y)

Date of assessment: /   /   (D/M/Y)

Clinical diagnosis

Inattentive subtype	(Please tick) ☐
Hyperactive-Impulsive subtype	(Please tick) ☐
Combined subtype	(Please tick) ☐
In partial remission (subthreshold symptoms plus impairment)	(Please tick) ☐
If no diagnosis, please give details of differential diagnosis:	(Please tick) ☐

	No. of symptoms	
DSM-IV diagnostic interview	Inattention	Hyper-imp
Childhood		
Adulthood		
Age of onset in years		
Pervasiveness criteria met	(Please tick) ☐ Yes ☐ No	
Impairment criteria met	(Please tick) ☐ Yes ☐ No	

Comorbidity

Mood disorder	Depression	(Please tick) ☐ Current ☐ Past
	Bipolar (specify subtype)	(Please tick) ☐ Current ☐ Past
	Other emotional dysregulation	(Please tick) ☐ Current ☐ Past
Personality disorder	Antisocial	(Please tick) ☐ Current ☐ Past
	Borderline	(Please tick) ☐ Current ☐ Past
	Other	(Please tick) ☐ Current ☐ Past
Substance abuse	Antisocial	(Please tick) ☐ Current ☐ Past
	Borderline	(Please tick) ☐ Current ☐ Past
Autistic spectrum disorder		(Please tick) ☐ Current ☐ Past
Dyslexia		(Please tick) ☐ Current ☐ Past
Tic disorder		(Please tick) ☐ Current ☐ Past
Anxiety disorder		(Please tick) ☐ Current ☐ Past
Obsessive compulsive disorder		(Please tick) ☐ Current ☐ Past
Eating disorder (specify anorexia or bulimia)		(Please tick) ☐ Current ☐ Past
Psychotic disorder		(Please tick) ☐ Current ☐ Past
Learning disability (IQ <70)		(Please tick) ☐ Current ☐ Past
Other disorder (Please specify)		(Please tick) ☐ Current ☐ Past